Bobby ~~

Thanks for all
the work you do
to educate ")

Love,
Regina
Nelson
7/24/17

W0009021

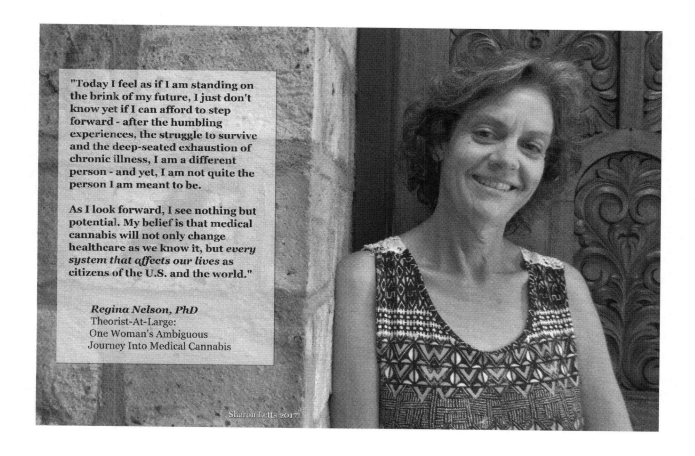

"Today I feel as if I am standing on the brink of my future, I just don't know yet if I can afford to step forward - after the humbling experiences, the struggle to survive and the deep-seated exhaustion of chronic illness, I am a different person - and yet, I am not quite the person I am meant to be.

As I look forward, I see nothing but potential. My belief is that medical cannabis will not only change healthcare as we know it, but *every system that affects our lives* as citizens of the U.S. and the world."

Regina Nelson, PhD
Theorist-At-Large:
One Woman's Ambiguous
Journey Into Medical Cannabis

Sharon Letts 2017

I published my first book, (*Theorist-at-Large: One Woman's Ambiguous Journey into Medical Cannabis*), in 2015. In it I shared that this academic journey has been "...a journey of a lifetime! Like nothing - NOTHING - I ever expected!" At that time, I had just resumed my studies after a medical leave of absence but I am thrilled to have met the deadline I set in Chapter Six of that book; to complete my Ph.D. journey in 2016!

And, the journey continues to be like nothing I ever expected!

This book isn't designed as a non-fiction text but is my dissertation in its entirety, as approved by my Union Institute and University Dissertation Committee: Dr. Michael

Raffanti, Dr. Jennifer Raymond, and Dr. Beryl Watnick. I am thrilled to be sharing it in a published form with those who've been champions on my journey and the many participants in my research.

To anyone who actually purchases it: *I thank you from the bottom of my broke little heart!*

This particular study was six long years in the making. I began my studies in Ethical and Creative Leadership January 3, 2011 and successfully defended this dissertation on December 2, 2016. For at least the last two years of academic work, I struggled with how best to conduct this research. For me, as a patient, much frustration (in addition to still being a criminal) is still associated with the process of obtaining a medical cannabis recommendation. Along this crazy journey this social scientist stumbled upon explaining cannabis use and targeting dosing for specific patients and illnesses in ways supported by science. My work had begun to help bridge the communication gap between patients and the medical community, as well as help patients new to cannabis understand why, how, and when it can be an effective treatment.

Yet, I have been denied a medical cannabis recommendation many times by physicians entangled in institutional policy, those completely ignorant on the subject, or ones unwilling to listen to my needs and experiences. These experiences combined with those shared with me by patients and doctors across the country only fueled my desire to expose the many ways medical cannabis programs marginalize those who participate in them. In the end, as you will read, the study's participants demonstrate the social significance of this project - and they do so in ways I could not have done through autoethnography. I am proud to have been a vessel to share their stories in a manner that will have social impact.

Thank you for supporting me along this crazy journey!

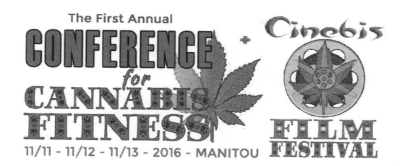

The First Annual
CONFERENCE for CANNABIS FITNESS
Cinebis FILM FESTIVAL
11/11 - 11/12 - 11/13 - 2016 - MANITOU

Cinebis Film Institute
is pleased to congratulate Dr. Nelson
on her Ph.D. in Ethical Leadership!

She proved to be an *integral* part of the historic proceedings which took place in Manitou Springs City Hall (including pressing live rosin onstage, thank you Emerald Fields + Apothecary Extracts) in autumn, 2016.

Another big thanks to the Manitou Springs City Council for the presence of mind and *ethical leadership* to provide their citizens with an opportunity to educate themselves about their own endocannabinoid systems! Also to Rocky Mountain Glass for the oil rig that commands place of pride on her variously arrayed dining room dab station!

The First Annual Conference for Cannabis Fitness + Cinebis Film Festival was one of the very last speaking appearances Regina Nelson made before very successfully defending her doctoral dissertation on December 2nd, 2016. That's the research you hold in your hands now. Again, Doctor, *Congratulations!*

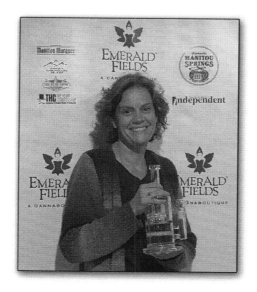

Dr. Regina Nelson on the Cinebis 2016 red carpet

Also from Regina Nelson, PhD.

- Theorist-at-Large: One Woman's Ambiguous Journey into Medical Cannabis
- The eCS Therapy Companion Guide (aka The Survivor's Guide to Medical Cannabis, 2018)
- Talking To Your Doctor/Patient About Medical Cannabis

Much of the information regarding the endocannabinoid system (eCS) or the use of cannabis as medicine are referenced from Regina Nelson's *The eCS Therapy Companion Guide*, available on Amazon, Kindle, in local bookstores, and at www.MyECSTherapy.Org. Also available, *Theorist-at-Large: One Woman's Ambiguous Journey into Medical Cannabis*, Dr. Nelson's first book! Ask your local independent bookstore to carry them all!

The Medical Cannabis Recommendation

An Integral Exploration of Doctor/Patient Experiences

By

Regina Nelson, Ph.D.

Edited by Michael E. Browning

~ planting a seed for cannabis education worldwide ~

Copyright © 2016, 2017 Regina Nelson, Ph.D., Integral Education Press
All rights reserved. www.IntegralEducationAndConsulting.com, Boulder, CO 80301
Second edition: Revised May 2017. Integral Education Press
First edition: December 31, 2016. The eCS Therapy Center

Editing, Book Layout & Cover Design: Michael Edward Browning
Author Photos: Sharon Letts

Printed in the United States of America. No part of this book may be used or reproduced in any manner whatsoever for financial gain without written permission - except in the case of brief quotations embodied in critical articles or reviews, OR as individually required by the book's owner to facilitate this important conversation within their own families and health care teams.

Integral Education Press and The eCS Therapy Center titles are available for special premium and promotional uses, and for customized editions. For further information, please call our Publishing Department at 1-720-767-2047.

Library of Congress Cataloging In-Publication Data
Nelson, Ph.D., Regina.
    The Medical Cannabis Recommendation: an integral exploration of doctor/patient experiences / Regina Nelson, Ph.D.
153 p. cm. "Cannabis Medical Research"
ISBN 13: 978-0-9758900-3-5
ISBN 10: 0975890034

Table of Contents

Abstract

This study seeks to better understand the experiences of doctors and patients as participants in state-run medical cannabis compassionate care programs. It specifically seeks to understand the program participant experiences with the medical cannabis recommendation process. An improved understanding of these experiences viewed through an AQAL framing helps us gain knowledge pertinent to future research in leadership, public policy, healthcare. As well it may have other academic applications. Examining whether system participants experience transformative learning may also provide information relevant to future educational structures. In the battlefield of the War on Drugs, when engaging with compassionate care programs, physicians and patients must contend with the polarities of state policies that conflict with the Controlled Substances Act (CSA) that bleed into all other aspects of a life. An integral methodology was applied to a narrative inquiry of 32 physician and patient participants. By assessing common and differing narratives through an integral lens (Wilber, 2000a), while grounding experiences in the All-Quadrants, All-Levels (AQAL) theoretical frame, a developed understanding emerges. Participants describe how the inter-objectified public and institutional policies (Lower Right Quadrant) affect the cultural (Lower Left Quadrant), relational (Upper Right Quadrant), and subjective consciousness (Upper Left Quadrant). Participant narrative highlights many factors that contribute to the marginalization of a growing population of chronically and terminally ill American citizens. However, participant narrative *also affirms that patients and physicians engage in transformative learning experiences.* Findings here will guide future research, educational initiatives, and assist with normalizing the use of cannabis.

Dedication

For all my grandchildren, those I adore now and the generations to come. Your future is reason enough. Daniel, Rachel, BreAnna, Stephanie, Timothy, and Bryan: each of you as individuals have inspired my life's journey in many ways. I am truly blessed to be your mother.

Acknowledgements

This Ph.D. journey has been so much more than I ever bargained for and I know it could not have been accomplished without a great deal of dedication, love, and support from many.

Billie Jo Holt and Gerald Nelson, my parents, as well as Nancy and Jack, my extra-parents, all empowered me to learn more - always *more*. Having four strong, loving people behind me has made life's challenges easier; this is no exception. They, like my children and grandchildren give me reason each day to continue forward though they may not have understood my journey or process, they loved and supported me through a rough ride.

A HUGE thank you goes to Michael Browning for assisting me through the final stages of formatting, editing, and publishing. Our creative collaboration will continue to be awesome! Many thanks are also extended to Bill Tobin and Mark Pedersen, who each played a part in my life and learning in an amazing way.

When I arrived at my first residency and was welcomed by The Cohort 10, I knew I'd have brothers and sisters to support my journey - and what a journey it's been for us all! So many willing shoulders to cry on, many a critical peer-review to ponder, and diverse perspectives to contemplate. Each member of The Cohort 10 has made an imprint upon my life. Thank you! Individually and collectively you encouraged me to develop as a person in ways I could never have comprehended when this program began. My scholarly efforts will always reflect a bit of Ezekiel Dukes, Carter Beavers, and each of us that stepped forward together in January 2011 for an adventure none of us could have imagined. To my many other cohort brothers and sisters, please know I am grateful for the gifts you've shared with me. Each of you played an amazing role in this journey.

Finally, no scholar can succeed without the support of academic leaders like those I've found at Union Institute & University. Dr. Toni Gregory imprinted my achievements by inspiring me more than she ever realized. The integral connection and understanding of Dr. Michael Raffanti is reflected in my work. He continuously encourages me to continue forward despite life's obstacles and reminds me often that more research follows this achievement. Dr. Jennifer Raymond has been a mentor since my first term and is an example of academic leadership that I hope to replicate as I move into academics. Though Dr. Beryl Watnick joined my committee late, her input and encouragement have been priceless. Thank you for supporting my academic journey at Union Institute & University!

Chapter One

Introduction

This study explores the medical cannabis recommendation process through the narratives of physicians and patients who have experienced it. This study seeks to better understand the experiences of doctors and patients as participants in medical cannabis compassionate care programs. It specifically seeks to understand their experiences with the medical cannabis recommendation process. An improved understanding of these experiences viewed through an AQAL framing helps us gain knowledge pertinent to future research in leadership, public policy, healthcare, as well it may have other academic applications. Examining whether system participants experience transformative learning may also provide information relevant to future educational structures.

The history of cannabis prohibition, public policy, and the process of medical cannabis recommendation are critical to developing an understanding of the importance of this issue, as well as the experience of participants in medical cannabis systems. Gaining a better understanding of this contextual issue will aid to improve social and public policy affecting current system participants. This chapter begins with an examination of the state-level medical cannabis policies and programs and the federal Controlled Substances Act.

Examining the Controlled Substances Act

Historians suggest that *cannabis sativa* was a predominant agricultural crop, food, and medication for thousands of years before its eradication in 1937, at the hands of Harry J. Anslinger, the appointed head of the U.S. Treasury Department's newly formed Federal Bureau of Narcotics (Herer, 1998). Demonized and criminalized since the late 1930s, *cannabis sativa* or "marijuana" has become a very misunderstood food, medicine, and agricultural crop. Scientific and medical researchers like Dr. Lester Grinspoon (2010), Dr. Donald Abrams (2013, 2016), Dr. Vincente Di Marzo (2014), and Dr. Raphael Mechoulam (2015) and many others have repeatedly and publicly stated that if the *cannabis sativa* were discovered today, given what we know about the endogenous cannabinoid receptor system, everyone - doctors, researchers, pharmaceutical companies, the media, and the public - would become well informed of its benefits because it would be heralded as a "miracle drug of a sort" (Mechoulam, 2015, ICRS). Despite the Shafer Commission's (1972) recommendation that "[T]he criminal law is too harsh a tool to apply to personal possession [of marijuana] even in the effort to discourage use...," President Richard M. Nixon urged Congress to pass the Controlled Substances Act (CSA) in the early 1970s to stymie illicit drug use across the United States. The CSA continues to classify *cannabis sativa* and all its phytocannabinoids as a Schedule I Controlled Substance.

The CSA categorizes drugs into five schedule groups, which are determined by the medical acceptance, abuse potential, and ability to produce dependence. The CSA also regulates the development and distribution of narcotics, stimulants, depressants, hallucinogens, anabolic steroids, and certain chemicals used in the production of illegal drugs. The CSA classifies *cannabis sativa* as a Schedule I drug with a "high potential for abuse" and "no accepted medical use," in the same schedule as drugs such as heroin, LSD, and ecstasy. Meanwhile, oxycodone and methadone, the most commonly abused prescription drugs and leading sources of opioid overdose deaths, are Schedule II drugs; implying that these drugs are less dangerous than cannabis though unlike opioids, it cannot induce a fatal overdose in and of itself. *Cannabis sativa* is non-toxic and its CSA classification unjustified since patients in twenty-eight (28) U.S. States have access to it for medicinal use (Nelson, 2015).

Establishing the CSA also combined existing federal drug laws, and more importantly, the nature of federal drug law policies. It expanded the scope of federal drug and law enforcement with regard to controlled substances. Michelle Alexander's text, *The New Jim Crow Law: Mass Incarceration in the Age of Colorblindness* (2012), provides a well-researched and startling look at the nation's escalation into a "War on Drugs" that citizens often experience as a war upon our own people. The enactment of the CSA and the classification of *cannabis sativa* as a Schedule I Substance is integral to public policies (LR), social beliefs (LL), education (AQAL), and many other influential convictions.

In contrast to other Controlled Substances, THC (Δ9-tetrahydrocannabinol), the prominently active phytocannabinoid, principal compound responsible for "euphoria", and reason for CSA appointment, is known to have a low level of abuse and its ability to produce dependence is also substantially lower than many nutritional supplements that remain unscheduled, like St. John's Wort (Nelson, 2014). The inclusion of *cannabis sativa* on the CSA encompasses all the plant's phytocannabinoids. This means that phytocannabinoids like cannabidiol (CBD), cannabichromene (CBC), cannabigerol (CBG) and many others are also restricted from research, education, and distribution despite growing scientific evidence that supports the medicinal use of these cannabinoids in conditions as broad ranging as Alzheimer's disease to Post-Traumatic Stress to Infantile Seizure Disorders. If one considers the substantiated facts related to cannabis and its phytocannabinoids, it should instead be classified as an essential nutrient - a safe and non-toxic essential nutrient at that (Nelson, 2015). Legalization advocates, lobbyists, historians, and even some physicians, were touting the medicinal benefits of cannabis use long before scientists discovered the endocannabinoid system (eCS) in 1988 (Mechoulam, 1988).

The startling evidence of the eCS and the plethora of resulting scientific evidence that has followed - despite CSA restrictions - has failed to morph the public dialogue about cannabis use from harmful, illegal substance to low-risk, non-toxic, potential health therapy or simple nutritional supplement for most, if not, all human beings. Nor, has public or professional education been a focus of policymakers. In short, the prohibition of cannabis has failed to become an issue of public health, in large part *because* of its CSA Schedule I status. The nation's patchwork of medical marijuana policies was neither designed nor implemented using public health lenses, even though these programs are typically assigned to state public health departments. Instead, these policies have been created by politicians and activist organizations that continue to promote the prohibition of cannabis, *except for* limited and restricted access for only the most vulnerable and ill citizens. The controversy and stigmatization surrounding this issue seem to counter significant scientific evidence that is a factor in the doctor-patient relationship and the recommendation required to participate in a medical cannabis program.

Science confirms that cannabis is a public health issue, which affects all citizens. The endocannabinoid system (eCS), named after the *cannabis sativa* plant that led to its discovery, is perhaps the most important physiologic system involved in establishing and maintaining human health (Petrocellis, De Grazia-Cascio and Di Marzo, 2004). Scientific research describes the eCS as an *endocrine system*, more recently as perhaps the body's *primary* endocrine system (McPartland et. al., 2006). Endocannabinoids and eCS receptors are found throughout the body: in the brain, organs, connective tissues, glands, and immune cells. The eCS is responsible for multifaceted actions in our immune system, nervous system, and the body's organs. It is literally a bridge between our body and mind. The eCS performs different tasks, but the goal is always the same: *homeostasis*, the maintenance of a stable internal environment despite fluctuations in the external environment (Nelson, 2015).

Public Health: What is it?

As defined by the World Health Organization, public health refers to, "all organized measures (whether public or private) to prevent disease, promote health, and prolong life among the population as a whole. Its activities aim to provide conditions in which people can be healthy and focus on entire populations, not on individual patients or diseases. Thus, public health is concerned with the total system and not only the eradication of a particular disease."

Further, the World Health Organization (WHO) describes the three main functions associated with public health:

1. The assessment and monitoring of the health of communities and populations at risk to identify health problems and priorities.
2. The formulation of public policies designed to solve identified local and national health problems and priorities.
3. To assure that all populations have access to appropriate and cost-effective care, including health promotion and disease prevention services (Public Health, WHO, 03/28/15).

Public health professionals at WHO or organizations like the Center for Disease Control (CDC) try to prevent problems from happening or recurring through implementing educational programs, recommending policies, administering services, and conducting research. Although a large part of public health is promoting healthcare equity, quality, and accessibility; public health also works to limit health disparities by considering the systemic causes and effects (WHO Website). Public health departments play a vital role in educating medical professionals and the public as new illness, products, and policies affect the masses.

The simple fact that every human being has an eCS should warrant public health status and legitimize medical cannabis programs. Sadly, however, our public health leaders and policymakers have failed to consider the scientific evidence; not only has the CDC and WHO failed to get involved in medical cannabis policy efforts, they - along with groups like the National Institute of Health (NIH) or the National Institute on Drug Abuse (NIDA) - forsake the responsibility to share important cannabinoid science with the public or educate medical professionals. As witnessed by repeated failings to remove cannabis from a State's List of Controlled Substances; every medical cannabis policy in the U.S. fails to incorporate this important knowledge. Simply put, policymakers are not considering medical cannabis from a public health perspective because the public health organizations refuse to become involved in discussion regarding a Schedule I substance. Unfortunately, this includes those assigned medical cannabis programs on the state-level, which doctors and patients may participate in.

Instead medical cannabis policies have been written and supported by lobbying groups, like National Organization for the Reform of Marijuana Laws (NORML), Americans for Safe Access (ASA) or Marijuana Policy Project (MPP). Thus far, these organizations develop medical cannabis policies from language used in initiatives that repealed alcohol prohibition nearly a century ago and have highly prohibitionist language (Pacula, Hunt and Boustead, 2014). Each of these organizations has also neglected to consider the public health needs of the citizenry they represent because they view the issue through prohibitionist lenses (Nelson, 2012). From quadriplegic Ashley Weber's unlawful eviction from Section 8 Housing (2012) to the loss of TANF benefits for medical cannabis patients in the State of Colorado who fail a urinalysis due to detected THC (2015) to the removal of Daisy Bram's children by Child Protective Services in California (2013), the consequences for medical cannabis patients are still steep under prohibitionist state policies that conflict directly with the federal CSA. These conflicts impact our social systems, including things like social services, healthcare, law enforcement agencies and every single person who seeks assistance or needs support from them, including doctors and patients.

Study after study confirms that the social stigmatization and criminalization of cannabis use are far more harmful than the actual use of cannabis itself (O'Brien, 2013; Nutt, 2010; Nelson, 2014 and 2015). Though the point of every cannabis policy has been *access* for the sick and vulnerable, demand already far exceeds supply. True access is limited to those who can qualify for a state program and *afford* to access medicine through the legal market. This requires a recommendation for medical cannabis and a lengthy registration process. Many still rely on the black market because they have been denied access, cannot afford, or do not qualify through the "legal" system. Others are afraid to join a marijuana registry. Since not all states require patients to register, it is difficult for scholars to access the magnitude of issues such as these. However, if every human has an eCS, then all humans are affected by these oppressing outcomes, particularly those at the center of the system: doctors and patients.

Doctor-Patient Relationships

Cannabis users have been criminalized, marginalized, and stigmatized for more than seven decades. As a society, we are having a hard time escaping these offensive social constructs and forming new ones; ones in which all humans have an eCS and can benefit from *cannabis sativa* holistically, as can our earth and society. Perhaps nowhere is this more noticeable than in the communication between doctors and patients. In contrast to public health officials, clinical professionals like doctors and nurses, focus primarily on treating individuals after they become sick or injured. However, they rely upon public health departments and institutional policies, as well as pharmaceutical sales representatives, to keep them informed of new policies, consumer alerts, product scams, vaccination information, and so on. With public health departments assigned medical cannabis programs not taking a leadership role beyond regulation, education languishes, the public remains confused, physicians fear entering discussions, and patients suffer in the margins.

Scholars have only recently begun considering the issue of medical cannabis and the social ramifications of the compassionate care policies millions of patients now rely upon as a portion of his or her healthcare system and for which physicians are the gatekeepers. Though few studies exist, recently, a team of Canadian researchers (Ziemianski et. al., 2015), published an educational needs assessment survey, which considered input from more than 500 physicians that begins to explore this issue. The researchers found that patients are far more likely to initiate the discussion about medical cannabis than his or her physicians and that physicians feel they have insufficient information and "lack guidance on the topic."

However, the greatest obstacle to medical cannabis recommendation was shown to be a physician's belief that patients are not actually seeking cannabis for medical purposes, but for recreational ones (p. 49). Given that this outcome corresponds with findings where patients report "a lack of trust by health care providers" and suggest that "it is due to the stigma associated with cannabis as an illegal recreational drug" as found by Bottoroff et. al. (2013), as well as the Hathaway et. al. (2009, 2010) studies. This more in-depth look at this issue demonstrates how these failings affect those in the system, specifically, the physicians who are providing medical cannabis recommendations and the patients receiving them.

In the United States, the clear majority of physicians are connected with or directly employed by our nation's hospital and clinic systems tying them all directly to federal funding through programs like Medicaid and Medicare, Veteran's Benefits, or even research funding (NIH, NIDA) and numerous private health insurance companies. All of whom are required to comply with the CSA by instituting zero tolerance drug policies, which prohibit the use of Schedule I substances.

Budget conscious administrators afraid of funding loss, combined with physicians who have not been formally educated about the eCS or the use of cannabis, implement policies meant to protect the organization, but which fail to recognize that every single patient is negatively impacted by the inability to recognize the public health implications of this issue. In fact, it is commonplace for healthcare organizations to forbid physicians from engaging in the recommendation process. The Schedule I status of cannabis is the primary reason for these policies. No hospital wants to put federal funding or insurance contracts at risk.

In large part, because this issue has not risen to the level of *public health crisis*, public and professional education has not become mandatory. As the gatekeeper for a medical cannabis recommendation, a physician cannot "prescribe" *cannabis sativa*. Instead, the physician evaluates whether a patient qualifies for the program provided in his or her state. If in agreement, the physician "approves" of the patient's use of cannabis under the designated guidelines set by the state by *recommending* medical cannabis.

Policies vary considerably but typically require a physician to attest to:
- ✓ verification of a qualifying medical condition
- ✓ the exhaustion of conventional treatments, sometimes including life-threatening surgeries or experimental pharmaceutical regimens
- ✓ a physical exam, may or may not be required.

Irrespective, some form of medical recordkeeping or specified state-required recommendation form must be completed. Typically, though not always, this information is provided to a designated public health department.

As described in "Untangling an Egregious Social Error: The Case for Medical

Cannabis Public Health Policy" (Nelson, *Integral European Conference, 2016*) vulnerably ill patients are often circumscribed to marginalization simply for seeking a treatment (which was commonplace in recent human history). Only 80 years ago, *cannabis sativa* was the primary tool in a physician's kit, so to speak. As marijuana became criminalized and hemp eradicated, physicians, much like farmers, had not yet made the connection between the new social scourge of smoked marijuana. In 1937, only 27 pharmaceutical products were approved within the U.S.; a full third of those contained cannabis. As well, as it was prominent among traveling salesmen's products, and what we would now call over-the-counter remedies (Nelson, 2015). Physicians did not understand that the eradication of marijuana would affect their ability to treat patients with *cannabis sativa*. Nor could farmer's explain the eradication of one of our nation's top producing agricultural crops: hemp or *cannabis sativa*.

In fact, in 1939, then New York Mayor, Fiorello LaGuardia, an outspoken opponent of the 1937 Marihuana Tax Act, commissioned the New York Academy of Medicine to consider the medicinal benefits of *cannabis sativa*. The LaGuardia Commission's findings were discounted as "unscientific" by Anslinger himself. Medical research continues to support cannabis as a non-toxic therapy, much as the LaGuardia Commission reported in 1944, (Herer, 1998) despite Anslinger's protests and the continued criminalization of the plant (Booth, 2015; Fine, 2014).

This extended prohibition of cannabis has also had an enormously negative impact on our understanding of the eCS and the phytocannabinoids from the *cannabis sativa* plant. Schedule I status restricts clinical research, much less any attempt at disseminating a public health message. Our global scientific community is just beginning to understand the eCS and how cannabis works synergistically within the body. As of now, there are few medical school courses that offer education on this vital endocrine system. Neglecting to educate physicians on the eCS has a significant impact on future patients' health. The public expects medical schools to educate about the nervous or immune systems. The eCS is a part of these systems that is being ignored. Justice as fairness, as well as human consciousness, requires we reevaluate cannabis as a public health issue and begin the normalization process to restore it to society. Considering the communication between physicians and patients is strained at best when it comes to medical cannabis recommendation, it seems a vital place to begin the normalization process.

The first part of this process is understanding the knowledge and experiences of doctors and patients (and the objective of this study). This study seeks to better understand the experiences of doctors and patients as participants in medical cannabis compassionate care programs. It specifically seeks to understand their experiences with the medical cannabis recommendation process. An improved understanding of these experiences viewed through an AQAL framing helps us gain knowledge pertinent to future research in leadership, public policy, healthcare, as well it may have other academic applications. Examining whether system participants experience transformative learning may also provide information relevant to future educational structures.

Scientific Evidence

Schedule I status hinders research and has discouraged human trials over the last 80 years. However, there is ample evidence - 25,000 plus studies - that suggest cannabis may prevent disease, promote health, and prolong life among the entire human population; the very tenants of public health. Currently, more than 100 academic and pharmaceutical company derived studies are published monthly that relate to new knowledge of the eCS functioning, or phytocannabinoid or synthetic cannabinoid interactions. This field of science is growing, yet this information is not being communicated to physicians or the public.

As mentioned earlier, organizations like WHO and CDC, or even State Public Health Departments that are assigned medical cannabis programs, neglect to adequately educate the public or health care providers about the eCS. The state-level compassionate care programs do not provide information vital to understanding how patients use, dose, and experience medical cannabis therapies. Simply put, they do not administer these programs like other public health initiatives: H1N1, vaccines, HIV/AIDS, birth control, or numerous other issues considered vital to public health that bring awareness to both medical professionals and the public. Instead these programs, simply regulate and manage enormously bureaucratic and marginalizing programs that disappoint those they are meant to serve.

Existing laws and policies only allow physicians to approve or certify a medical cannabis recommendation. Unlike a prescription drug, the doctor cannot control the number of purchases, what is purchased (e.g., % THC or other cannabinoid content), where it is purchased (e.g., dispensary, patient grown and processed, or black market), or the route of administration (e.g., inhale smoke or vapor, ingest an edible, or apply topically). The hesitancy to provide a recommendation can easily be correlated, at least in part, to the failure to provide physicians and patients with adequate education and information on which an informed decision about cannabis therapy can be made. How will the patient use cannabis? How much should they use?

Further stymying doctor-patient communication in this context, is the common consensus among medical professionals that advocacy is a poor substitute for the dispassionate analysis of evidence-based medicine (EBM). Seemingly in majority opinion, physicians agree that popular vote should not prevail over scientific evidence in deciding whether cannabis is an appropriate medicinal agent for the masses. In Konrad and Reid's 2013 study, "Colorado Family Physicians Attitudes Toward Medical Marijuana," the researchers found only 19% of the 520 physician respondents even believed physicians should be recommending cannabis for patients; as many as 46% did not support recommending cannabis at all. An exploration of the reasons for this belief seem vital to patient care and success of these programs, especially since Colorado's medical program is often used as a model for other states. This study begins to illuminate how others have changed beliefs and accepted medical cannabis as an issue of diversity. By assessing narratives that describe how doctors and patients as participants in compassionate care programs are experiencing the medical cannabis recommendation process, we can learn ways to improve these services.

Schedule I status has had an enormously negative impact because it in effect prohibits the medical establishment's preferred model, the randomized clinical trial (RCT). Funding is simply not allocated for projects that consider the medical efficacy of a Schedule I substance in humans. While Western allopathic physicians are devoted to the RCT, public health is not as biased and relies on disciplinary and interdisciplinary methodologies to consider health from much broader perspectives than EBM and the RCT.

Physicians have become comfortable with the RCT model, in large part because this is how they learn about and understand new drugs that come to market. The role of the pharmaceutical sales representative is to provide an overview of this type of information on new drugs to physicians. Though GW Pharmaceuticals (2013, 2014, 2016) has RCTs in progress in the United States and has RCT data for products Sativex and Epidiolex, these data are not distributed by public health departments or physicians. It is not considered directly relevant to the products patients purchase in regulated dispensaries. This means even vague parameters to using the compound in question, (therapeutic dosing level, risks and side-effects, etc.) are not made available to physicians - or to the patients undergoing therapy.

On the other side of this relationship, when researchers asked patients how they make health-related decisions, among the top answers were; access to information, assertiveness, sufficient time since diagnosis, education, good interactive relationships with nurses and physicians, [and] encouragement by nurses and physicians to participate in health-related decisions (Say, Thomason, & Murtagh, 2006). Unfortunately, because the traditional medical community holds so little knowledge regarding cannabis therapy, patients can rarely rely on these important factors to help them. Thus, from a public health perspective, informing the medical community and public is of utmost importance. However, how are we to inform them if we do not have RCTs or tools they will recognize?

In attempting to see the broadest picture, an interdisciplinarian must look beyond disciplined boundaries and into what scholar Allan Kaplan (2005) calls the "invisible spaces." Doctor-patient conversations about the recommendation of cannabis occur in these spaces; between individuals who are products of cultural and social values and beliefs. Interdisciplinarity gives us the means to look between disciplines and into the invisible spaces where real world problems exist and require creative solutions. Considering the doctor-patient relationship and the influencing factors that are engaged in a discussion about the recommendation of medical cannabis from multiple perspectives enhances understanding of the subtleties in play, as this study establishes.

Medical Cannabis Recommendation

   More than half of U.S. States (28 of 50) and the District of Columbia have adopted some type of "Compassionate Care" policy that allows for restrictive access to cannabis for a defined population of terminally or chronically ill patients. Estimates place the number of recognized medical cannabis patients at over 2,000,000 across the nation (ProCon.org). Over two million U.S. citizens whose treatment relies little on accepted medical knowledge, but heavily on anecdotal information shared amongst communities of patients, social media, internet news, and even some mainstream media. In 2013, NIDA projected as many as 19.8 million Americans used cannabis within the past year. Since the use of cannabis is a health-related activity given its ability to supplement the eCS, these users can be classified as cannabis patients to some degree, though they are not recognized as such. Further, the United Nations (2014) places the global number of cannabis users at nearly 160 million. It seems likely that many more people engage in cannabis therapy than estimated, but currently most patients find themselves in a disorienting dilemma, when it comes to discussing a medical cannabis recommendation with a personal physician. This means many remain hidden in the black market, are forced to pay a medical cannabis evaluation center, or simply go without a potential therapy.

   In obtaining a recommendation outside of primary doctor-patient relationships, like through a medical cannabis evaluation center, the patient's desire to avoid stigma takes precedence. It takes courage to stand against social convention. Bottoroff, et. al. (2013) explore the patient perspective in their article entitled "Perceptions of cannabis as stigmatized medicine: a qualitative descriptive study" stating,

   Even more problematic from a human rights perspective is the potential for discrimination in the healthcare system, where individuals fail to receive appropriate assessment and treatment for a health condition because of being labeled as drug dependent or a "pothead". In this context, patient-provider consultations become focused on extraneous issues, such as addiction and one's moral fiber, rather than the larger concerns of symptom management and the underlying pathology of illness. Amid this preoccupation resides an uneasiness and lingering doubt that cannabis for therapeutic purposes (CTP) use is contrived and manipulative, whereby cannabis is masking, and in many cases adding to, the individual's and societal problems. This discourse threatens the trust essential for a caring patient-provider relationship and may disrupt future care-seeking behaviour by patients as well as the delivery of efficacious treatments by healthcare providers. (p. 8)

Terminally and chronically ill people often have difficulty sharing voice (UL). The results of this study provide an improved understanding of the many influential factors that are engaged when a recommendation for medical cannabis enters a discussion between doctor and patient.

Through social media, patients share testimonials of doctors refusing to enter a conversation about the use of cannabis with them. Others have reported physicians walking out of a consultation; physically showing his or her blatant refusal to discuss a vital issue. Not every patient is rebuffed as this study shows, but sadly, most patients in medicalized states who thought the enactment of a medical cannabis policy would help bridge this communication gap have found that it has not. As with other studies, most of the registered medical cannabis patient participants did not receive the actual medical cannabis *recommendation* from a personal or specialty physician. Instead they found the services of a "pot doctor" or a medical cannabis evaluation service. The burgeoning industry is but a reminder of interdisciplinarian, Stanley Fish's (1989) observation that,

> "Knowledge [can be] frozen in a form supportive of the status quo"

(p. 100).

Across the country, a work-around system has emerged that forces patients to often pay large sums for an evaluation and recommendation from a physician they may or may not ever see again. Recent medical school graduates deep in student loan debt and retirees fill a gap that should not exist. When *Fortune* magazine (February 11, 2016) reported that the medical cannabis industry could approach $7 billion in 2016, it failed to mention that this enormous amount of revenue does not include ancillary cannabis-related businesses (non-dispensaries, non-cultivation, non-program licensed), like evaluations centers.

Substantiating this assertion, Mikuriya et. al. (2007) found that in California - among physicians operating practices integrating cannabis therapy - more than 95% of the patients were "self-medicating" prior to the receipt of his or her recommendation. This finding led the panel of researchers to conclude that the physicians were really "approving" the use of medical cannabis as opposed to "recommending" it (p. 41-43). In short, the primary support proffered by the physician for cannabis therapy is the recommendation; rarely is it supplied along with education, consultation, or referral to a social service agency. These models still do not exist, in large part because this issue is not treated as a public health concern.

However, the physician's recommendation is a cornerstone requirement of compassionate care policies serving as a gateway for a patient to have safe, legal access and a small modicum of rights associated with the possession and use of cannabis. Instead of gaining acceptance within the medical establishment and community, largely because cannabis remains a Schedule I substance, this work-around system is becoming institutionalized. The reasons for its existence are examined in this study and discussed by participants in Chapters Four and Five.

It is an act of leadership for a patient to stand against social conventions challenging healthcare providers with a new proposal or their own embodied knowledge; an experience sought in desperation after conventional therapies have failed to provide relief. As well, it is an act of leadership for physicians to educate and act in ways that support the use of cannabis as a public health issue, while still faced with the reality that our social policies, and oftentimes institutional policies concerning the medical use of cannabis are inadequate. Patients are forced outside their normal doctor-patient relationship by ignorance and fear of stigmatization (Bottoroff, 2013). Understanding how doctors and patients as participants in compassionate care programs are experiencing the medical cannabis recommendation process from an AQAL perspective increases knowledge. As well, it helps us understand that system participants are undergoing transformative learning as a result of these experiences.

Even though twenty-eight (28) U.S. States and the District of Columbia have enacted some medical cannabis policy scheme (ProCon.Org) rights granted to recognized medical cannabis patients vary considerably and do not extend beyond a state's borders due to the federal Schedule I status. Conditions under which a patient may qualify for a medical cannabis program also vary considerably. California is the most compassionate state allowing 'any condition that may benefit' the patient as attested to by a physician. Since 1997, this particular caveat, included because of the eCS, has caused the most federal interference in California's medical marijuana program. In comparison, Illinois has thirty-nine (39), "qualifying conditions" under which a patient may register as a medical cannabis patient, with the recommendation of his or her "bona fide" physician (i.e. M.D. or D.O. only). This means that evaluation centers, the legitimate, but costly work-around for patients afraid to enter the discussion or refused a recommendation by his or her personal physician, are highly discouraged in Illinois. The few that have cropped over the first year, during the program's implementation, have been highly scrutinized and several have already been fined or closed. The idea is right; patients should be able to discuss a medical cannabis recommendation with a personal primary and specialty care physician without fear of stigmatization or loss of status. As well, physicians should have information about the eCS and the use of cannabis to share with his or her patients. This however is not the reality medical cannabis patients experience currently as this study's participants share in Chapters Four and Five.

The lack of attention to this issue solidifies a black market because it places legal access at a point of unaffordability or is too cumbersome for those who could most benefit from it. Certainly, not all, but many Illinois hospitals and clinics have already instituted medical cannabis policies that prohibit attending or resident physicians from recommending cannabis - following the example of other U.S. states that medicalized earlier. Citizens seeking a recommendation believe most have already implemented these policies because they are so common, so they don't even inquire. This study demonstrates the result is a lack of power and authority on the part of both physician and patient as it relates to this issue.

Dominant public narratives are clear and citizens who experience using cannabis illegally understand they must, "contend with prejudicial labels and reefer madness sentiments that culturally endure" (Hathaway et. al., 2011, p. 463). For patients that come to consider medical cannabis in a new pilot program like that in Illinois, far fewer have the type of experience described in Mikuriya et. al. (2007), which was conducted in California. In Illinois, both doctor and patient are ingrained in the social myths and stigmatizing behaviors associated with cannabis use having little knowledge about the program or how others may experience medical cannabis nationally. A patient must muster the courage to enter a discussion knowing that the physician may change the way they view them, as well as be unsupportive or uneducated about the subject matter. Participants share that this experience is not unique to Illinois but problematic across all medical cannabis state programs.

Unlike predominant "stoner" stereotypes, studies consistently confirm that medical cannabis patients are likely to be located, with lesser or greater degrees of social visibility, "all over the map" of actors and institutions (Hathaway et. al., 2011; Pedersen, 2009; Smucker Barnwell et. al., 2006, Earleywine, 2002). U.S. demographics suggest that most are male and over the age of 40, (www.norml.org) but by its own demographic report, the Illinois pilot program is attracting women, over the age of 60, with fibromyalgia, who've run out of conventional options (IDPH Report, June 2015). Patients who anticipate support from a "bona fide" doctor but seldom find it given the abhorrent statistics.

In an essay entitled, "Perceptions of the Dominant Discourse as Experienced by Female Cannabis Patients" a study participant described this type of marginalization from her vantage point as a Registered Nurse (Nelson, 2015).

To "continue a career in medicine - a career I really love," she considers it "vital" that she conceal her [medical cannabis] status from others especially, "co-workers and hospital administration" to avoid stigmatization, loss of status, and/or loss of employment. Expressing her fear of stigmatization, she states, "I do not tell people I work with that I am a medical marijuana patient - they would do a random drug test on me and I would be fired and not be able to get a job in this town again." Her main concerns include that "co-workers" will "assume my judgment is impaired, even if I have not been using marijuana," or that "I would be considered [lazier] than others." She believes,

"...especially in my last position, in the supervisory

17

position I had, the knowledge [that] I am a medical marijuana patient would have hindered my ability to do my job because of the stigmas associated with marijuana use. So, I don't tell anyone I work with I am a patient. I am still very much a 'closeted' patient because it is just too big a career risk."

On the other hand, the participant states that she and her co-workers ("the doctors and nurses") have had conversations as "experienced professionals that are out there seeing what it can do for patients...how much better patients can control their symptoms [specifically, like pain] with cannabis at times." She maintains these conversations "never get personal," because the only time she shared the "news of receiving my patient card" with a "trusted colleague," she was admonished by her "friend." She was told, "he had lost faith in me and my ability to return to school to be a Nurse Practitioner," because "now all you'll do is sit around and smoke pot all day." This participant felt an immediate *loss of status* and *marginalization* from this interaction - with someone she "knew understood this medicine can be good for patients like me - who'd even suggested I try to get my card." Experiences like this or even just the fear that this type of experience might occur, oppress cannabis patients causing them to fear and hide from marginalization. [It kept this study participant from engaging with her personal physicians and "forced me to drive two hours and pay a small fortune to see a pot doctor."] Engaging in a workplace known for both pre-employment and random drug-testing creates a hostile work environment for cannabis patients. This nurse shares that there are not others "willing to admit [their patient status] in the workplace" or "discuss this seriously or in-depth." She was very frightened and arguably marginalized (Nelson, 2015, p. 168).

If an educated medical professional believes that to supplement her eCS, she must forfeit job security and assume "much risk" for "challenging the medical

establishment by choosing a non-toxic, and safer alternative to prescription drugs."
(Nelson, 2015, p. 123) then how do other medical professionals and patients experience
the recommendation process? Gaining an understanding of how others have
experienced the medical cannabis recommendation process will assist public health
leaders tasked with educating physicians and the public. This type of knowledge also
opens a path to improved public and institutional policies.

In large part, people lack understanding in this arena because few researchers
have considered the subject of medical cannabis from the perspective of those
experiencing these new systems. To date, most research in this area falls into the
categories of scientific research (on the eCS, endogenous cannabinoids,
phytocannabinoids, synthetic cannabinoids, or substance abuse) and public policies
(arguments for or against the prohibition of cannabis). Few academic articles consider
those using cannabis except as a substance of abuse, and even those, rarely consider the
patient's narrative and actual experience (Reiman, 2014; Ogborne, 2000; DeWitt, et. al.,
2000; Hathaway et. al, 2011; Nelson, 2014 & 2015). As a new and emerging social
phenomenon, this domain is ripe for research of all kinds. Given the increasing
complexity and ubiquitous nature of our modern world, the cannabis movement is but a
microcosm of our greater society. Much like the HIV/AIDS crisis was once gripped by
the lack of focus from a public health perspective (Andriote, 1999), research from a
variety of frames, like this integral study, highlight the most prominent problems in our
broken social systems through the lens of this public health issue.

The Researcher

Throughout my Ph.D. studies at Union Institute and University, I have
experienced significant health problems. My personal journey as a medical cannabis
patient began in 2011 when I moved from Texas to New Mexico *as a medical cannabis
refugee* during my second semester of coursework. After studying the medical effects
and potential benefits of medical cannabis, I desperately hoped that it would provide me
with some relief. I had received diagnoses for three "qualifying conditions" within the
State of New Mexico with significant medical records as evidence; yet, I still had a

difficult time obtaining a medical cannabis recommendation. My own doctors were prohibited from providing recommendations by their medical institutions.

In the end, it took me three months to save the $250 fee a local Physician's Assistant required to certify my medical cannabis recommendation. After an extensive review of my medical records, he approved and completed the required medical cannabis recommendation form but he was unable to provide me with any details relevant to dosing medical cannabis for my conditions. As I left the consultation, two D.E.A. Officers in full uniform held the office door open for my exit. I was more than a little unsettled and disturbed by the exit experience. Two months later, I finally received my medical cannabis card and felt relieved to be acting within the laws of my state. However, I also came to find that the dispensaries I had awaited visiting were unable to provide any details relevant to dosing medical cannabis either. About the same time the physician's assistant contacted me to share that an investigation by licensing authorities had been launched following a tip by the New Mexico State Health Department that he was recommending medical marijuana for qualifying patients.

When I relocated to California in 2012, my second medical cannabis recommendation experience was less dramatic given there was no D.E.A. interference. Then again, there also wasn't much medical knowledge or experience shared beyond a tele-med physician (apparently on break from his job in a busy Emergency Room) asking me if I did indeed have the listed qualifying condition and if I had any questions about using cannabis. Unfortunately, though he asked if I had questions, the physician was unable to answer a single one of those I brought forward. For instance,

"Are there better ways of using cannabis medicinally?"

or "Am I using the right amount?" In short, I paid nearly $100 for the pleasure of having a physician sign a piece of paper, so that I might comply with the law in the State of California for six months. Combined state and federal law enforcement had pushed to close nearly every dispensary in San Diego where I was living. I was left on my own to figure out how cannabis might work best for me, plus, I had to several drive hours north for any hope of finding legal access to the specific products that I needed.

By 2013, in Colorado, the medical cannabis recommendation process wasn't as difficult as it had been in New Mexico, but it wasn't as easy as it had been in California either. A wonderful, holistic physician took time to review my full history and ask me many questions about my symptoms and diagnoses, but as with the other physician's who'd recommended medical cannabis for me, he was unable to answer questions about dosing and using cannabis. Another $175 in fees for a medical appointment outside my normal health care system, but for a year I could comply with the laws of my new home state.

When it came time to renew my medical cannabis registration in Colorado in 2014, I took a chance speaking with three of my personal physicians: my primary care doctor, plus a hematologist and a gastric specialist. Each had medical records in hand that provided evidence that medical cannabis was aiding in my recovery, thanks to one of my New Mexico physicians who'd followed my progress closely; however, not one was willing or able to complete the medical cannabis recommendation form required for my renewal. Two cited clinic policy prohibiting doctors from recommending cannabis for any patient. The third, the hematologist, is also an oncologist, who does recommend medical cannabis for cancer patients. However, I was not being treated for cancer, so she stated that she could not provide a recommendation renewal. In asking the doctor, "What do you know about the endocannabinoid system and its role in my anemia?" She collected my charts very angrily and stated "I don't know anything about that but what I do know is that I won't sign your renewal." She left the room with a slam of the door leaving me alone and stunned. Five minutes earlier, she had asked me if I felt like I was dying, "because you are" but she would not spend even a few minutes listening to how cannabis was helping me cope with the symptoms she knew were killing me slowly and painfully. If I hadn't been two years into this topic of study and endowed with embodied knowledge, I might have given up. Instead I paid another $150 to an evaluation center physician for a renewal, so that I might comply with the state's laws another year.

During these experiences, the frustration I felt as a patient was closely linked to the external and internalized stigma that I faced. These experiences, as well as the relief I'd found using medical cannabis, prompted me to act. The eCS Therapy Center, a national non-profit organization, is the outcome. As C.E.O. and President of the Board of Directors, my leadership has focused on peer-to-peer education programs, accredited curriculum for the medical cannabis industry and medical professionals, and research related to the experiences of medical cannabis patients. This work involves me with patients and medical professionals across the globe.

It has also exposed me to the stories of many of the participants prior to the conception of this project. Though I was not familiar with the recommendation experience of participants prior to interviews, I was not shocked to hear that many of the patients had similar experiences to my own. Although the sharing of patient experiences brings awareness to our plight, including the narratives of physicians helps readers understand the complexities that create obstacles for both participants in the medical cannabis recommendation conversation. As this study demonstrates, it is vital to consider the experiences of doctors and patients as participants in these new social systems. Future social and public policies must gain a better understanding of these same experiences so that appropriate change and better policies can be implemented.

This study explores how doctors and patients as participants in compassionate care programs are experiencing the medical cannabis recommendation process. To take a more comprehensive view of this situation, an integral methodology (along with its valuable All Quadrants, All Levels (AQAL) framework) was utilized in a narrative study.

The research questions were as follows:

1. How are doctors and patients as participants in compassionate care programs experiencing the medical cannabis recommendation process?
2. From an AQAL perspective what are participant experiences telling us?
3. Are participants undergoing transformative learning as a result of these experiences?

In this study, 32 participants shared their experiences to help address these research questions. This data was coded and sorted using Philosopher Ken Wilber's *Theory of Everything* (2000b) and its AQAL framework. Integral theory and the AQAL frame were built upon Koestler's notion of the holon construct. Koestler (1967) described this nested hierarchy, in which each whole is "both...and" as parts, as well as wholes, as a "holarchy." A holon is the "nodal point in a nested hierarchy...that can be seen and described in terms of its holistic and independent nature as well as part-ness and dependent nature" (Edwards, 2005, p. 270). People, whether patients or doctors, are individual holons, participating in roles, within a greater holarchy that is the context and the initiative they are enacting, in this case the conversation regarding the recommendation of medical cannabis. The AQAL model advances the notion that in looking at issues from a single quadrant perspective, conventional scholars, and even many postconventional scholars are missing the bigger picture.

AQAL discloses fundamental paradigms for conceptualizing social reality. As the frame of integral theory, it helps contextualize multiple truths; revealing the domain of validity of any theory - its truth *and* its limitations (Esbjorn-Hargens, 2009). Andrew Vickers and Anton de Craen (1999) state that,

"The illness belongs first of all to the person who is ill, the *patient's experience* is the ineradicable fact of medicine."

Yet, patients are also the texts to be examined, studied, and understood, even if they don't always read like a book (p. 9). Physicians are the readers of these texts, they read by understanding the signs and fitting them together into a recognizable, communicable whole, but every reader has habits, prejudices, and expectations, as well as, taken-for-granted assumptions, feelings, or values that may bias practices including communication and action.

This study finds the disconnect may lie in the morality of using an illicit (Schedule I) substance (LL, LR) as medication, failure of the patient to follow standard Western protocols (UR, LL, LR), or any number of other beliefs, values, or cultural concerns, as will be examined in Chapter Four and Five findings. The AQAL frame allows us a view at the conjunction of individual and collective phenomena between doctor and patient, allowing the truth of participant experiences to be revealed, contrasted, and examined.

Particularly, this exploration also sought to determine if participants, both patients and physicians, engage in *transformative learning* experiences because of personal experiences engaging in this disorienting dilemma. In Chapters Four and Five patient participants discuss experiences (that accompanied the journey from chronically or terminally ill patient to medical cannabis leadership) and physicians (who have shifted personal beliefs about the use of cannabis from substance of abuse to medicinal agent) share his or her transformative learning experiences.

Chapter Two discusses the integral frame and the study's methodology in greater detail.

Chapter Two

Literature Review

This theoretically informed, narrative inquiry seeks to understand the various factors that affect the doctor-patient experience when a medical cannabis recommendation enters the conversation. Integral Theory and Transformative Learning form a two-part conceptual framework from which narrative data was explored. The use of narrative theory is a pedagogical approach that provides a reflective and interpretive methodology for making sense of stories and experiences shared by participants. In this case, the researcher gathers the raw data of the experience with the aim of promoting a deeper and more coherent understanding of the factors affecting doctors and patients through analysis of the collective interview data. How are doctors and patients as participants in compassionate care programs experiencing the medical cannabis recommendation process? And, what, from an AQAL perspective, are participant experiences telling us? Finally, have participants experienced transformative learning because of these experiences?

Integral Theory

In Chapter One, Wilber's *Theory of Everything* (2000b) and it's All-Quadrants, All-Levels (AQAL) framework were identified as an analytic lens. Integral theory is built upon Koestler's notion of the holon construct. Koestler (1967) described this nested hierarchy, in which each whole is "both...and" as parts, as well as wholes, as a "holarchy." A holon is the "nodal point in a nested hierarchy...that can be seen and described in terms of its holistic and independent nature as well as part-ness and dependent nature" (Edwards, 2005, p. 270). In other words, physicians and patients are individual holons participating in roles (collective holons) within a greater holarchy (AQAL) that are doctor-patient relationship experiences; as well as the context they are acting within, like a conventional or alternative health care conversation. The complexity of this relationship, as well as individual, cultural, or social values held about the context of the conversation, lends to the value of an AQAL frame. Donna Ladkin (2010) uses Merleau-Ponty's notion of "flesh," a construction "capable of providing a means for understanding the dynamic in between space" as appropriate for the AQAL frame. As this study reflects, this description is fitting, particularly when exploring the core of relationships such as the relationship that exists between a doctor and a patient. The inclusive AQAL framework calls attention not just to what is happening for each individual or system, but what is happening in the spaces in between (Volckmann, 2012, p.22).

The AQAL is a model and the foundational structure of *integral theory*. It is a method of integral pluralism that attempts to integrate as many valid systems of knowledge as possible into an inclusive, metatheoretical framework (Esbjorn-Hargens, 2009). AQAL has two axes: the horizontal axis denotes a continuum between interior and exterior realities and the vertical axis signifies a continuum between individual and collective realities. Together, the four quadrants are the fundamental domains in which change and development occur in individuals and collective groups. It is useful to consider integral theory as a system of analytical lenses that can provide a more comprehensive picture of social, political, or cultural circumstances and possibilities. For these reasons, it was well-suited for this narrative inquiry.

AQAL Overview

UL Interior Individual Consciousness Subjective Learning I	**UR** Exterior Individual Behavioral Objectified Learning We
LL Interior Collective Cultural Intersubjective Learning It	**LR** Exterior Collective Social Interobjectified Learning Its

The AQAL model effectively supports an integral approach, as the interaction of its dimensions produces the fundamental domains through which developmental change occurs. An integral approach maintains that understanding any social phenomenon requires at least two fundamental dimensions of existence be considered. The quadrants can and often are causally related, such that changes in one produce changes in the others (Astin and Astin, 2001, p. 72; Nelson, 2012). As participant narrative demonstrates the four dimensions are interconnected and irreducible.

Considering integral approaches to healthcare, physician Dr. Joel Kreisberg (2007) believes the value of the AQAL frame is in arguing that clinical decisions may be considered from each of these four perspectives, "providing a unique integrated meta-perspective that cannot be reduced into any of the four fundamental perspectives" (p. 370). As AQAL demonstrates, "there may be a multiplicity of valid answers to questions and that integrating contrary or conflicting perspectives may offer more complex, subtle, or complete answers (i.e., both/and)" (p. 370). Integral methods "involve attention to individual development and behavior, organizational cultures, and organizational systems in relation to socio-eco-political systems in which they operate" (Volckmann, 2012, p. 3).

Taking this approach, illuminates the obstacles, such as social stigma, as well as collectively and individually held beliefs at play in the doctor-patient relationship. As well, it provides insight into how these prominent beliefs or values change, as described by participants.

The AQ or "all-quadrant" aspect of AQAL, encompasses "the I, we, and it dimensions (or self, culture, and nature; art, morals, and science; first-person, second-person, and third-person)" (Wilber, 2000b, p. 138). Development of the "I" recognizes the interior, subjective space where each person, whether patient or doctor, values the importance of exploring one's own health and well-being. This is where one becomes integrally conscious of one's knowing, doing, and being in all aspects of personal or relational endeavors. Addressing how one has been denied life expression would also be an aspect of this type of development.

The principle of "We" recognizes the importance of intersubjective spaces, like where doctors and patients come together and share worldviews, beliefs, priorities, and values related to improving healthcare. For doctor-patient relationships to be fully represented in this space a focus on understanding what the other person (doctor, patient, family, other healthcare professionals, or others) is expressing or not expressing is needed. This is where miscommunication can easily occur, especially when an emotionally-charged conversation engages a disorienting dilemma, like the medical cannabis recommendation.

The principle of "It" recognizes the importance of the individual exterior or objective space, where a therapy plan is developed and integrated, for instance. Between doctor and patient, "doing to" and "doing for" occurs in this arena (Beck, Dossey, and Rushton, 2011, p. 75). This space includes patient education, evaluation, interventions, and life practices that "interface with and enhance the success of traditional medical and surgical technology and treatment" (Beck, Dossey, and Rushton, 2011, p. 75-76), including the recommendation of medical cannabis therapy.

The "Its" principle recognizes the systems and structures of the exterior collective or interobjective spaces where physicians and patients join the wider healthcare systems and institutions. Reflections of the influences of healthcare and public policy systems are revealed through stories of lived experience (as this study exhibits).

To see the whole picture, each of the four quadrants must be explored in relation to one another. In understanding the life experience of an individual doctor or patient, the UL or internal, subjective meaning-making, and UR or objective actions and behaviors are relevant. As well the context of LL or objective systems and LR or collective cultural and meaning-making systems impact both parties and often differently. In this exploration, an integral understanding was developed from a narrative analysis on the subjective meaning to individual doctors and patients (UL); observations/ demonstrations of individual behaviors within the doctor-patient relationship were shared narratively (UR); each participant discussed tools and processes to be used on the collective level (LL) and the impact of federal CSA status, as well as other institutional policies and practices (LR). The inquiry also reveals many social and cultural characteristics that affect the conversation about medical cannabis recommendation (LR/LL). Additionally, it reveals narratives specific to transformative learning experiences.

Narrative analysis allows the researcher a view of these phenomena, as well as of the spaces in between or the relation among the quadrants (AQAL). Using Wilber's AQAL model, one can study the perspective of each quadrant from their complex interconnected relationships and as a holonic model, in that each quadrant is equally important to the whole. Esbjorn-Hargens (2009), describes, integral theory as "a powerful framework that is suitable to virtually any context and [which] can be used at any scale" (p. 2). He finds that it "allows a practitioner to select the most relevant and important tools, techniques, and insights because, "it organizes all existing approaches to and disciplines of analysis and action" (p. 2). This researcher experienced this during data analysis, as will be shown in Chapter Four.

LR: Institutions, Systems, and Processes

State medical cannabis public policies fall squarely within the LR quadrant as does the federal CSA. State compassionate care policies have been a primary focus of advocacy groups related to patient access for "safe, legal" cannabis medication that is "taxed and regulated," as noted in Chapter One. Interdisciplinary Professor, Michael Schwartz (2013) finds, "Politics is the mode of engagement called forth by justice as reverberating through the LR quadrant such that the other three quadrants are sensed through the moral lens of a politics of justice-fairness (p. 171)." In relation to public health policy, this means system approaches must answer Rawls' call of *justice as fairness*.

In an integral sense, public policy must move out "of political power-as-dominance into political power-as-empowering;" as well, there must be "an eco-politics (where humans are only one species amongst many), a family-politics (where one has an ever-changing set of roles as one ages), a state-politics (which brings forth questions and issues of governance and public deliberation) and so on (Bashkir, 1993, p. 171)." Policymakers seem to pay little attention to cannabis patient needs outside of the LR quadrant and attention within the realm is primarily focused on regulation and restriction, failing to engage in public or professional education. However, the doctor-patient relationship and the participants' experiences are affected by this realm as compassionate care policies endorse the physician as gatekeeper for medical cannabis access via the recommendation process. This remains outside of conventional medical systems, such as those the doctor and patient relate within, particularly, in this case, U.S. healthcare systems.

As described in, "Untangling an Egregious Social Error: The Case for Medical Cannabis Public Health Policy" (Nelson, *Integral European Conference*, 2016), issues related to the doctor or patient experiences come from individual and collective intersections with the LR quadrant. Perhaps, most negatively impacting the doctor-patient discussion about the recommendation of medical cannabis is the fact that no public policy mandates education for either medical professionals or the public. This means the physician is not adequately informed about either the eCS or the use of cannabis and neither is the patient. For patients seeking more information and the opportunity to engage in cannabis therapy this presents a conundrum. Do they attempt this conversation or do they avoid it? Given that Mikuriya, et. al. (2007) found more than 95% of the patients were "self-medicating" prior to the receipt of a recommendation, it is reasonable to believe the majority avoid the conversation unless they anticipate acceptance. Patient participants in this study further confirmed this belief. Further, participating patients rarely report being directed toward cannabis therapies by a personal or specialty physician. Physicians seem to also be avoiding these conversations as supported by Bottoroff et. al.'s (2013) findings and physician participants of this inquiry. Although the federal CSA's Schedule I status of *cannabis sativa* is a direct factor, there are more nuanced understandings and additional aspects, which participants shared and are reviewed in Chapter Four.

In Chapter One the new phenomenon of medical cannabis evaluation centers was discussed, work-around to primary care physicians and patients engaging in this primarily administrative process. These models have become familiar to the public in many medicalized cannabis states and provide the majority of medical cannabis recommendations for requesting patients. However, as was also noted, Illinois is among the first to require a "bona fide" doctor-patient relationship as a condition of approval for the medical cannabis program. In other words, medical cannabis evaluation centers, where patients assume they can avoid stigmatizing behaviors and receive a certain amount of support, are not acceptable based on LR policies. For patients in this newly medicalized state there appear to be several observable responses:

1. accept the risk of stigma by asking a personal physician - believing the outcome may be negative and fail to result in a medical cannabis recommendation
2. adamantly avoid the conversation while continuing, beginning, or considering black market alternatives
3. desperately search for a new doctor after receiving a denial
4. incur out-of-pocket expenses by visiting an evaluation center, or
5. remain unaware that cannabis therapy may be an option for you or a loved one

For physicians, fear about recommending a Schedule I Substance are real but often misunderstood. For many, these fears may prevent them from educating themselves or from considering cannabis a viable therapy for a requesting patient. For Illinois patients, it has taken nearly two years to register less than 9,000 patients (IDHP, June 2016 Report).

LL: Culture and Shared Values

Common language, signs, and symbols that are understood and shared with others characterize the LL quadrant. If we are to successfully rescript cultural beliefs about what it means to be a cannabis user or to recommend or use cannabis as a medical therapy, this realm requires reflection. Until the taboos, rituals, and shared meanings about cannabis use are demystified, patients and doctors, will continue to suffer. This is especially true given that cannabis use is not yet considered a public health issue. Although, CNN's Dr. Sanjay Gutpa (CNN, "Weed" Series, 2013, 2014, 2015) has admitted his earlier ignorance about cannabis and the eCS, apologizing publicly and educating others via mainstream media about its benefits, with no public or professional education requirements in place, myths and misinformation plaguing both sectors, the ability to shift social perspectives is a daunting task. Educating millions of global citizens can only be achieved if cannabis patients are willing to share private voices publicly, particularly with medical and other service providers, as well as public leaders. Additionally, in order that both parties might understand the issue better, patients also must learn how this affects physicians, sharing stories with physicians would begin to fill this gap, yet many patients avoid engaging in these types of conversations. This academic understanding of this phenomenon, from both the doctor and patient perspective, is valuable to the future of medical cannabis programs and those who participate in these systems.

Given the Schedule I status of cannabis (LR), continuing myths, and misinformation about its use and effects, as well as the failure to educate medical professionals or the public about the science that supports its therapeutic benefits; these outcomes are not surprising. The social status of cannabis users, even those who only use medicinally, is much as Hathaway, et. al. (2011) find,

"that [cannabis] users might alternatively be viewed on a normative continuum that has shown signs of shifting in the theorized direction of greater

32

sociocultural acceptance (or indifference) of the practice, while retaining vestiges of social disapproval that contribute to maintaining a 'culture of control,'"

as espoused by Philosopher, Erving Goffman (Hathaway, 2011, p. 46). In other words, the use of cannabis as medicine has not been normalized in the sense Goffman (1963) proposed though as a society - collectively - we appear to becoming more accepting of the practice, as witnessed by the compassionate care policies now blanketing the U.S. However, as participants share, much more action - particularly in the realm of education and research - is necessary.

Physicians and patients are both immersed in a culture of control as participants in healthcare systems. Physicians, as experts, are viewed as *controllers* of therapies; while patients, non-experts, are *receivers* of prescribed therapies. "When health practitioners are viewed as experts who tell you what to do, individuals become passive participants, blindly following protocols without taking authorship of their own lives" (Zucker, 2011, p. 133). The request for a medical cannabis recommendation impacts the doctor-patient relationship directly in this space. Marginalization occurs when patients are rebuked for requesting treatment challenging the norm or the expert. Study participants discuss issues of the withdrawal of support, loss of status, or lack of understanding from a primary or specialty care physician, in oppressing terms.

Goffman further describes *normal* as incorporating standards from wider society and meeting others' expectations about *what we ought to be.* The concept of stigma is therein a device that ensures the reliability of the interaction order by punishing people who do not conform to moral standards. Some cannabis patients note a considerable cultural shift in opinion toward cannabis users, and state politicians respond by pushing forward restrictive, prohibitionist policies trying desperately to satisfy growing public opinion that cannabis should at least be made available for medical use. In contrast, others fear being exposed as cannabis patients with internalized (UL) and institutionalized (LL) stigmatization notably affecting his or her quality-of-life. Despite research to the contrary, a majority of public policymakers refuse to budge from the

33

stance that as a Schedule I drug, cannabis has no medicinal value. To a large degree, acceptance of the practice of using cannabis appears to be related to the extent of one's understanding - or ignorance - of the scientific or anecdotal evidence rather than the virtue of one's convictions about cannabis use, whether one is a doctor or a patient. The findings of this study help develop an understanding of these perspectives, including how some experience a change of belief that could have significant cultural impact.

Tam Lundy (2011) argues that integral theory provides us "an effective map to support thinking, practice, and evidence-gathering ... [and allows the] capacity to address the full complexity of human experience in an increasingly complex world because it is a meta-framework" (p. 46). An integral evaluation of a metanarrative, where basic commonalities and relationships become more apparent among the multiplicity of perspectives (or even traditions) of doctor-patient relationships provides effective, and sometimes surprising, results.

As Lundy describes, the "result is a map of reality that incorporates both subjective and objective dimensions of life, in individuals as well as collective contexts" (p. 46). In short, AQAL connects the dots between theory and evidence (p. 50).

UR: Body and Interpersonal Behaviors

Professors John Astin and Alexander Astin (2001) substantiate that this quadrant has been "the hallmark of modern, biomedical science and practice for much of the 20th century" (p. 75), for as a bodily experience physical health is within this quadrant. Stigmatization affects individuals with a variety of medical conditions (HIV/AIDS, hepatitis, post-traumatic stress, chronic pain conditions, and cancer, among others); arguably, cannabis patients with these conditions are *dually stigmatized* (Bottoroff et. al., 2013; Nelson, 2014). While the original principles of EBM emphasize the role of patient preferences (UL), cultural values (LL), and system issues in healthcare decisions (LR), critics of EBM suggest that it only recognizes research originating from an empirical perspective (LR).

Integral Methodological Pluralism (IMP), as presented by Scholar and Physician, Dr. David Petrie (2011), has the potential to improve EBM by expanding the breadth of medically usable knowledge without sacrificing depth or rigor of truth validation. Petrie supports the finding that there is opportunity to improve the practice of medicine through the integration of the insights of IMP into the principles of EBM. In the article, *AQAL: Beyond the Biopsychosocial Model*, E. Baron Short (2006) also explores IMP as an appropriate methodological approach to study the nested hierarchical levels of human development, including the psychological (UL) and cultural (LL) domains. Short finds,

"The AQAL model emphasizes the need for the physicians to continually transform personal awareness in order to best serve their patients"

(p. 137).

Stigma is internalized in the UL quadrant, but enacted through individual behaviors (UR), like those associated with either concealment or revelation. To more effectively handle complex issues, like medical cannabis, Esbjorn-Hargens (2009) elucidates, "[integral theory] systematically includes more reality and interrelates it more thoroughly than any other current approach" (p. 1). One may conclude that an approach that considers the UR quadrants relationship within the holonic AQAL frame has the potential to be more successful than the continuing biomedical focus on this singular quadrant. Integral medicine requires integral approaches; otherwise, cannabis patients will continue to be forced to evaluation centers that provide a less stigmatizing situation and environment, but one which comes with a steep price tag. In the end, both doctor and patient suffer from a failure to communicate adequately about the health needs of the patient.

Since health and behaviors are located within the UR quadrant, cannabis patients are adversely impacted by current public policies (LR) significantly in this domain. If cannabis use were addressed as a public health issue, the doctor-patient relationship would benefit, as would the public perception of patients using cannabis (LL). This would lessen the internalized fear many patients and physicians suffer (UL) that adversely affects relationships (UR). Per Kathryn Montgomery Hunter (1993), evidence based medicine "requires a bottom up approach that integrates the best external evidence with individual clinical expertise and patients' choice." Williams and Garner (2002) take this argument further stating, "The emphasis on hard scientific data tends to devalue sophisticated clinical expertise largely derived from experience and the detailed study of individual patients" (p. 71). In other words, the anecdotal information the patients choose to share or conceal. Yet, the EBM hierarchy (LR) is considered among the medical community to be the consensus opinion of care providers (LL/UR). For this reason, it is a dominant discourse re-enforcer within communities (LL). It also fails to address the medical experiences of patients who treat themselves outside standard western medical practices (LL), like medical cannabis patients. Given that patients embody far more knowledge about the use of cannabis than is currently contained in RCTs seems to escape the medical community. As well, this phenomenon marginalizes millions of people. Both patients and physicians participating in this study have suffered for pioneering in a new arena.

Face to face with a patient, a physician can know suffering only indirectly and subjectively; the same holds true of clinicians involved in RCTs or other clinical research. The signs they observe and the story of symptoms or side-effects a patient describes to them are simply data to be interpreted. "Thus, modern medical practice is founded on an arduous scientific education augmented by formidable diagnostic machinery, but interpretive skill is inevitably required for physicians to work even their everyday wonders" (Hunter, 1993, p. *xviii*). Diagnosis and treatment are a form of art doused in science. Understanding more about the complex communication between doctor-patients as it relates to this expanding arena of science is vital and has applications beyond the topic of medical cannabis.

UL: Personal Meaning and Sense of Self

The Upper-Left (UL) quadrant references the interior reality lived by a person. Theorist, Michael Schwartz (2013) describes the UL quadrant as "posited as the locus of the master or key hermeneutic arena of perspectives; or, in greater balance, the lens through which the other quadrants are seen, interpreted, and evaluated" (p. 169). This quadrant encompasses a person's subjective personal experience. Internalized guilt, fear, or stigma has effect on a patient's well-being and on both parties' decision-making in this quadrant. Hunter states,

"Medicine's goal is to alleviate present suffering. Although it draws on the principles of the biological sciences and owes much of its success to their application, medicine is (as it always has been) a practical body of knowledge brought to bear on the understanding and treatment of particular cases"

(p. *xi*). From an individual perspective, a patient seeks more from a visit to the doctor than the taxonomy of a malady. As an example, patient participants of this study seek an UR relationship that includes co-decision-making as discussed in Chapter Four.

The AQAL frame discloses fundamental paradigms for conceptualizing social reality. Psychologist Mark G. Edwards (2008a) elucidates, "These integral lenses tap into the worldviews that structure our interpretations of reality" (p. 181). The interior-exterior dimensions identify worldviews and social constructs that define a focus on either the subjective or the objective aspects of reality (LL/UL). Further, Edwards claims:

This integral indexing of worldviews and their associated pathologies makes available a means for identifying the patterns by which we construe or misconstrue our pasts, interpret our present and enable or disable our futures (p. 184).

The findings of this study demonstrate the effects on participants in all four quadrants and will provide a clearer understanding of this complex issue.

Transformative Learning

For doctors and patients, the recommendation of cannabis is a paradigmatic shift. Theorist, Jack Mezirow (1991, 2000) led the field of transformative learning research offering a theory of learning that is "uniquely adult, abstract and idealized, grounded in the nature of human communication" (Taylor, 1998, p. 173). The theory of transformative learning has been a focus of research in medical education, cooperative extensions, health education, educational administration, and communications; as a theory, it is relevant to this project.

Transformative learning theory is developmental in nature, it explores learning as the "process of using a prior interpretation to construe a new or revised interpretation of the meaning of one's experience in order to guide future action" (Mezirow, 1996, p. 162). The conversation regarding the recommendation of medical cannabis between doctor and patient might be described by Norman Denzin (1989), as an "interactional moment and experience which leaves marks on people's lives" (p.70), for just this reason. Certainly, many patients describe it this way; this study validates that physicians do too. Commons et. al. (1996) point out that during crisis points and "liminal" experiences, epiphanies have been shown to be a key factor in state development (Erickson, 1963, Commons et. al., 1996). In other words, those requesting or offering a medical cannabis recommendation may be at a gateway to a transformative learning experience. If so, what is it they learn from this conversation? Does this enact change within them?

Transformative learning has been found to be effective at capturing the meaning-making process of adults, particularly the learning process related to paradigmatic shifts (Mezirow, 1991, 2000, Cranton, 1994, Boyd and Meyers, 1998, Gregory and Raffanti, 2010). As described by Mezirow (1991), *a disorienting dilemma* can be a catalyst for change, and may affect a transformative learning process. As mentioned, the recommendation of cannabis, or a request for one, presents just such a disorienting experience for most patients and doctors. This narrative inquiry with an applied AQAL frame sheds light on the role of context (medical cannabis recommendation), the nature of the catalysts of transformative learning, other ways of knowing at play, the doctor-patient relationship, and provides a perspective of transformative learning that has not been explored academically.

In a review of transformative learning studies, Edward Taylor (1998) notes that there is little research about the possibility and process of transformative learning occurring in a particular context or as the result of a specific life event. He states,

> "More research about the nature of *learning experience* and how it informs our understanding of transformative learning is critical."

(p. 176). In this study, a narrative approach captured a retrospective snapshot of the participant's learning experience, increasing the understanding about this type of social phenomena. The challenge for this study was to separate out what was related to transformative learning from what was a product of normal development of an individual given this context. The developmental stages accompanying the AQAL framework guided the codifying process of potential transformative experiences, as discussed in Chapter Three and demonstrated in Chapter Four.

Engaging in relationships with others is an essential factor in the transformative learning experience (Taylor, 1998, 2016). Lisa Baumgartner (2002) provides some interesting insights about the nature of dialogue and relationships. She leads, *Living and Learning with HIV/AIDS: Transformational Tales Continued*, quoting Mezirow and stating:

> *Learning and development are intertwined, lifelong endeavors.*
> *Learning continuously reshapes people. Although some learning*
> *simply augments knowledge, such as learning a new version of*
> *a word processing program, transformative learning allows a*
> *person to become 'critically aware of one's own tacit*
> *assumptions and expectations and those of others and assess*
> *their relevance for making interpretations' (Mezirow, 2000,*
> *p.4). Individuals reevaluate their assumptions and gain 'a more*

dependable frame of reference...one that is more inclusive,

differentiating, permeable (open to other viewpoints), critically

reflective of assumptions, emotionally capable of change, and

integrative of experience' (Mezirow, 2000, p. 19 in

Baumgartner, 2002, p. 44)

Inherent in relationships is the engagement in dialogue with others, which is an essential aspect to transformative learning. Among people who were diagnosed HIV positive, Baumgartner found that social interaction and dialogue led to consensual validation (p. 46). In other words, "realizing they were not alone on this transformational journey" eased UL suffering by providing validation to personal experience, as discovered through communication with others (UR), other patients and physicians (p. 49). Dialogue between patients and physicians regarding the use of medical cannabis are highly personal and self-disclosing. This leaves both parties participating in a disorienting dilemma when it comes to the recommendation of medical cannabis. This thorough evaluation of both perspectives aids both parties by exposing barriers to this communication.

Particularly relevant to this discussion is Mezirow's (2000) "perspective transformation" theory. In short, this type of transformative experience helps one develop a new and more dependable frame of reference, "one that is more inclusive, differentiating, permeable (open to other viewpoints), critically reflective of assumptions, emotionally capable of change and integrative of experience" (p. 19). Other scholars have built upon the work of Mezirow (King, 2003, Cragg et. al. 2005) and offer insight into the transformation of meaning-making processes, "where participants retain their larger worldview (frame of reference), but their immediate beliefs or expectations (meaning schemes) may continue to change" (Taylor, 177). Paradigmatic shifts such as this are becoming more readily observed in the cannabis community among doctors and patients and were attested to by many of this study's participants. However, as Taylor elucidates, "the often-unquestioned celebratory nature of transformative learning and the overlooked negative consequences, both personally and socially, of a perspective transformation" must be considered as they relate to the issue of medical cannabis. Though transformative learning experiences are often linked to leadership development, a positive expression of the event, they may also be linked to negative consequences, like an exacerbation of post-traumatic stress for a critically ill patient, a negative expression of the same event, for instance.

Context and individual role play parts in shaping transformative learning experiences and have historically been overlooked in transformative learning theory (Clark and Wilson, 1991, Taylor 2016). Both prior life experiences and historical events have been shown to be contextual factors impacting transformative learning (Gregory and Raffanti, 2010; Baumgartner, 2002). This study aims to provide greater clarity to the context of the medical cannabis recommendation conversation, as well as the varying nature of perspective transformation as experienced by participants. The medium of narrative inquiry helps demonstrate the interplay between the personal and the social meaning-making of participants involved in the study. The personal (UL) and the social (LL/LR) are revealed in dialectical relationship. Researchers like Carolin Kreber (2012) and Liimatainen et. al. (2001) encourage other researchers to develop frameworks and coding schema that help identify the presence and/or levels of critical reflection among study participants particularly for those developing medical education research. The AQAL framework addresses these challenges with its meta-framework as demonstrated in Chapters Four and Five.

Imperative to transformative learning is finding ways to enact the new sense of social possibility that the change encompasses. For example, Elizabeth Lange (2004) found transformative learning "is not just an epistemological process involving a change in worldview and habits of thinking, it is also an ontological process where participants experience a change in their being in the world including their forms of relatedness" (p. 137). The relationship between transformation and action is supported by other scholars (Courtenay et al, 2000; Baumgartner, 2002; Garvett, 2004). For the reasons provided, and for the purposes of the proposed study, a transformative learning experience will be considered valid if a participant:

1. reveals a transformed view of themselves
2. demonstrates a commitment to help others understand the new perspective, and
3. validates an improvement in communication contributed to the transformation

Expanding the definition of diversity to any combination of differences and similarities is a jolt for those who have become accustomed to equating difference with conventional notions, like gender, race, or nationality. However, the use of cannabis is an issue of diversity and of social importance. AQAL provides a meta-framework from which shared language, ideas, and concepts may be generated so a theory may be formed. In addition, to gaining knowledge about doctor-patient interactions and forming a better understanding of the individual and collective dynamics at work, selected study participants engaged in the medical cannabis recommendation discussion process on several occasions; some successfully, some not. As a doctor or patient experiencing a significant change of mind, behavior, and actions the study revealed many had experienced transformative learning as a probable outcome of engaging in the recommendation process.

Narrative Inquiry

Scientific knowledge attempts to illuminate the universally true by *transcending* the particular. Narrative, on the other hand, attempts instead to illuminate the universally true by *revealing* the particular (Charon, 2006, p. 57). Educational Psychologist, Jerome Bruner (1986) was among the first to advocate for narrative ways of knowing in professional medical practice. Bruner observed that unlike analytical thinking, narrative "brings different insights and meanings to the "intense social interactions that often constitute patient care" (p. 13). He argued "narrative without analysis is naïve and analysis without narrative is meaningless" (p. 2).

Qualitative studies are often stereotyped as soft and subjective, in contrast to the hard and objective sciences, but narrative's soft data illuminates hard realities, as this study demonstrates. Physician and Qualitative Researcher, John Rich of *Healing Hurt People*, (Corbin, et. al., 2009) considers the impact of trauma surgery in young, black survivors of penetrating violence. His in-depth interviews give dramatic insight into the lives of socially marginalized patients. His findings also empowered participants "when a genuine interest in their lived experiences" was offered (Corbin, et al, 2009, p. 46).

Only a very small percentage of medical studies include this type of narrative data currently. While objective morbidity and mortality data characteristically remain faceless, narrative inquiry seeks not only to personalize, but also to engage with its research population through deliberate intervention. Narrative research is conducted with, not on, people. Narrative inquiry is desperately needed in the cannabis community. Exposing the issues obstructing medical cannabis programs, at least from the perspectives of the doctor-patient relationship, on which these programs depend is timely.

Kaplan (2002) suggests that, "We cannot simply struggle against the current status quo from within the paradigms which inform it; we must let go and move beyond" (p. 4). Narrative inquiry gives us the means to move beyond the status quo, to look between disciplines and into the invisible spaces where "real world problems" exist and need creative solutions. This is where the recommendation for medical cannabis lies: in a discussion, that is a real-world problem, lying in an invisible, and as yet, unexplored space.

Norman Denzin and Yvonna Lincoln (2003) argue, "Social research aimed at social improvement is not an inferior counterpart of "pure" social research" (p. 141). In fact, they suggest,

"Social change-oriented research, specifically action research, is the form social research must take if it is to achieve valid results, bring about useful social change, and reconnect universities to the larger society."

(p. 142). In not considering boundaries, which is at the heart of interdisciplinarity, researchers are free to break away from habitual ways of thinking and look at real problems with new eyes. The goal of the AQAL framework is to build a structure in the space betwixt and between disciplines that explores the whole in a way that validly disrupts the status quo. Together with qualitative research methodologies, integral theory seeks to answer these types of questions and offer an exploratory approach that unearths knowledge at the heart of the research question it poses.

The essence of narrative knowing is to frame and link interactions, like those between doctor and patient, into a plot or storyline. A story line provides a structure from which interactions or experiences may be understood by linking individual events (UR) to a larger whole (AQAL). Narrative knowledge is what one uses to understand the meaning and significance of stories through cognitive, symbolic, and affective means. This kind of knowledge provides a rich, resonant comprehension of a person's situation as it unfolds in time, whether in texts or in life settings such as medical appointments. Unlike scientific knowledge, through which a detached and replaceable observer generates or comprehends replicable and generalizable information, narrative knowledge leads to local and particular understandings about a specific situation by a participant (Bruner, 1986, p. 18-19).

This comparative analysis of the narratives of thirty-two (32) participants with varying lived experiences develops a more complete understanding of the social phenomenon of interest.

The narrative considerations of this study probe the intersubjective domains of participant knowledge and experience, specifically revealing aspects (AQAL) in the relation between doctor and patient regarding the recommendation of medical cannabis. Medicine, as an enterprise in which one human being (physician) extends help to another (patient), is always grounded in the intersubjective domain (UR, UL); however, the intersubjective is always affected by the objective (LL, LR), which is revealed through narrative. Medical practice, as well as the lives of patients and physicians, unfold in a series of complex narrative situations, including those between the doctor and patient, the physician and him or herself, the physician and colleagues, as well as patient or physician with family, friends, and cultural groups or greater society. Integral Theory is valuable to deconstructing the various experiences and helped the researcher code the data appropriately. Chapter Three will discuss narrative further as it describes this project.

Narrative in Medicine: Life Story

Research focused on medical education includes far more narrative inquiry than a clinical or EBM study; however, scholars are advocating for this method to spread more broadly into clinical arenas. Dr. David Petrie (2011), Professor of Emergency Medicine at Dalhousie University, elucidates:

> *Evidence-based medicine is an extremely influential movement within conventional medicine. When understood, and utilized appropriately it can significantly improve both the diagnosis and therapy for patients, leading to improved health outcomes. Unfortunately, however, although EBM recognizes the importance of system factors, patient preferences, and cultural values, it is not as strong at articulating how to assess evidence in these areas [therapy decisions made between doctors and patients]. In fact, the word* evidence *itself is often misunderstood to mean empiric evidence only (p. 10).*

Integral Methodological Pluralism (IMP) offers a potential solution to this limitation of EBM and its empiric evidence. An IMP-informed EBM, "recognizes evidence from all eight zones and the hierarchy of evidence" that exists within zones and not across zones (p.10). An IMP-informed EBM also provides a map, language, and methodologies to more clearly understand and articulate the role and impact of individual values and beliefs, relational issues specific to the doctor-patient relationship, influencing cultural values and perspectives, as well as health system values and perspectives with regards to clinical decision making and empathetic care (p. 11). This type of information is relevant and needed in the medical cannabis domain as this study makes evident.

In the conclusion of the article "The Shadow on Mammography: An Integrally Informed Paradigm Shift for Breast Cancer," Dr. William Argus (2011) notes that "organized medicine has failed to adequately control breast cancer despite its high-priority status and billions of dollars in research" (p. 23). He suggests that an alternative, integrally informed paradigm for breast cancer that looks at the whole person is needed. Narrative inquiry compliments this IMP process which, embraces "multiple perspectives in a way that honors human beings rather than reifying the disease" (p. 23). Argus supports a narrative inquiry "informed by the AQAL model" as an effective tool to facilitate developmental growth for patients, as well as physicians (p. 25). He points out that patients, as well as physicians, must also do the developmental work to fully understand how they embody illness and the treatment choices that they make (p. 24). A process of inquiry, informed by the AQAL model, that explores an issue, like the recommendation of medical cannabis, can facilitate that developmental growth. For this reason, the methodology employed in this study is rich in perspectives that must be shared.

In relation to integral psychiatry, which relies more extensively than clinical research upon narrative inquiry, Psychiatrist, E. Baron Short (2011) states,

> "Our story-making capacity is innate and matures with experience and complexity of cognition and self-identity. Our personal narratives have the potential to include the larger currents of life and the cosmos itself."

(p. 51). Integrally guided narrative inquiry exposes the implicit contexts of self and worldview that structure a person's experience. Life story is localized in the UL quadrant, but interpretation is influenced by UL and LL cultural perspectives, as well as LR social situations. Supported by Short's work,

> *A patient's narrative capacity is contextualized by dimensional*
> *complexity, whether represented as development lines of*
> *cognition (Piaget, 1977), ego identity (Kegan, 1998), or orders*
> *of consciousness (Kegan, 1995). The greater the reflective*
> *capacity of a person, the more complex a narrative can be*

woven. A person's implicit worldview, derived from culture,
and ultimate concerns often provide the underlying matrix of a
life story. Other experiential, cultural, and social systems
perspectives additionally influence an individual's narrative
complexity (Short, 2011, p. 52).

For these reasons, narrative inquiry provides insight into the various dynamics the doctor-patient relationship endures during a complex disorienting dilemma, like the recommendation of cannabis. How someone constructs a story is influenced by all quadrants of the lived experience. The life story perspective elucidates how assimilation or obliviousness of an increasingly complex body of knowledge or storytelling process impact one's experience.

The deconstructing of narrative data for this project revealed influencing factors from an AQAL perspective. These findings are shared in Chapter Four.

48

Chapter Three

Methodology

This study explores how doctors and patients, as participants in compassionate care programs, are experiencing the medical cannabis recommendation process. From an AQAL perspective the study is designed to help us understand how participants of these systems experience the medical cannabis recommendation process. As well, it examines whether participants are undergoing transformative learning because of these experiences. To take a more comprehensive view of this situation, an integral methodology, along with its valuable All Quadrants, All Levels (AQAL) framework, was employed in a narrative study that included 32 participants: 12 licensed physicians, either M.D. or D.O and 20 registered medical cannabis patients. Participants provided clear detail of how both parties are affected and the obstacles they must overcome. As one physician remarked, "There is a huge need for finding affordable providers who are willing to do this and not just sign a paper and say goodbye! Help with monitoring and observation and make it a real part of the patient's whole care system." But, how are doctors and patients experiencing the medical cannabis recommendation process? From an AQAL perspective what are participant experiences telling us? And, are participants undergoing transformative learning, as a result of these experiences?

Qualitative studies are often stereotyped as soft and subjective, in contrast to the hard and objective sciences; however, this study's narrative data illuminates' hard realities and internalized stigma and support Nelson's (2016) finding that medical cannabis policies and programs are not robust enough to address the real needs of patient populations or the physicians who support them. As this study finds, there are many areas that need to be comprehensively addressed for either party to successfully navigate a medical cannabis program. Chapter Five will discuss these findings in more depth.

For this study, using a "convenience sample" of participants was an effective option given the parameters of data to be collected (Remler & Van Ryzin, 2011, p. 141). John Creswell and Vicki Piano-Clark (2007) agree that convenience sampling is appropriate when selecting qualitative research participants, when the sample is based on specific purposes associated with answering a research study's questions, like specific knowledge or accessibility to the researcher. Given these parameters, the following criteria for selecting study participants was employed:

1. Evidence that the physician or patient has acknowledged him/herself as a medical cannabis patient or provider, i.e. public testimony of participation in the process or a transformative learning experience related to medical cannabis recommendation process
2. Accessibility during the data collection process to the researcher and
3. Informed, voluntary participation granted

In total, 50 potential participants were invited to take part in this project. Patients were notably more enthusiastic about participating than physicians. All 25 of the potential patient participants would have contributed but for accessibility during data collection to the researcher. In short, our schedules could not be coordinated. Of the 20 conducted patient interviews, 16 were accomplished by telephone; and 4 were performed face-to-face. Of the 25 physicians invited to participate, 12 interviews were conducted by telephone. Schedule coordination was expectedly more difficult; as well three of the physicians declined to participate as compensation was not offered to participants. In fact, no participant received payment for contributing to this study.

Internal Review Board (IRB) consent to participate in research was thoroughly reviewed with each participant *prior to the interview*; ensuring that each fully understood participant rights. In total 32 participants gave informed consent and participated in interviews. Though participants were provided an opportunity to withdraw consent immediately following the initial interview, no participant withdrew from the study. All participants were asked to review the transcript from the interview for correctness and given an additional opportunity to contribute to the project prior to data analysis. In total, 20 of the participants contributed additional data or clarified information contained within his or her transcript at that time. Further, all 32 participants were provided a rough draft of the study and requested to provide additional input. Nearly all participants (27 of 32) took this opportunity to provide final feedback to the researcher. All interviews were recorded for transcription by September 15, 2016, electronic means were deleted on October 31, 2016 and all related papers shredded.

Prior to beginning the interview, the researcher explained to all informed participants:

> *The focus of this study is on a particular context of the medical cannabis patient experience: specifically, the conversation between a physician and a patient regarding the request for a medical cannabis recommendation. The researcher is not requesting information about the use of cannabis prior to the legal recommendation of medical cannabis, but is seeking information particular to the access of a recommendation for cannabis under which you qualified (or provided support) in a U.S. State which provides a Medical Cannabis Program.*

This statement was included to assure that patients specifically, but physicians as well, understand that the use of medical cannabis or prior, potentially illegal use of cannabis, is not the focus of this study. As an added layer of protection for participants, only data regarding the recommendation of cannabis under a state-approved compassionate care policy was applicable for this study. However, despite the disclaimer patients (20 of 20) and physicians (4 of 12) commented on the personal use of cannabis, even if that use was illicit. As well, patient participants were asked to verify that they indeed are a registered cannabis patient in the state they reside and physicians were requested to provide the status of his or her medical license.

Participants

All 32 participants met the above criteria and were selected based on availability for an interview and follow-up given the schedule of the study. Using the AQAL frame and a narrative method helped reveal how both sets of participants attributed subjective meaning to inner (UR) experiences and reveals a view of his or her reality, as experienced across the quadrants (AQAL). Though participants were requested to recount personal experiences within the medical system (LR), specifically as it relates to the doctor-patient relationship (UR), most also reflected on relationships within family and social environment to clarify responses (LL/LR).

Physician Participants

The 12 physicians interviewed consisted of two females and 10 male physicians, with ages ranging from 32 to 74 years; meaning that recently licensed as well as retired physicians participated. Nine of the physicians were Caucasian and three were either of Hispanic or Indian descent. As mentioned, only M.D.'s (8) and D.O.'s (4) were placed in the physician category. A naturopath, non-M.D., non-D.O. also participated in the study, but her role was assigned as a patient, due to the parameters of the study, including that she is unable to certify recommendations; however, she is a registered cannabis patient. Additionally, four of the M.D.'s and a D.O. have notable research backgrounds and/or Ph.D.'s in specialties that include pain, obstetrics and gynecology, biophysical chemistry, and medical cannabis. Each of the 12 participating physicians is licensed to practice medicine in one of the following medical cannabis states:

Washington (1)   Oregon (2)   Colorado (2)

Arizona (1)   California (2)   New Mexico (1)

Illinois (2)   Nevada (1)

The physicians noted completion of medical school from the following institutions: University of Illinois, Washington State University, Texas College of Osteopathic Medicine, University of Missouri Columbia, John Hopkins, Yale Medical School, and Philadelphia College of Osteopathic Medicine. Only one physician noted that he has a related-degree and was employed in computer programming prior to attending medical school; however, two completed Ph.Ds. before attending medical school. The physicians are or have practiced in the following specialties: Palliative care, Family Practice, Integrative Medicine, Pain Management, and Holistic Medicine. Several hold Board Certifications: Integrative Holistic and Complementary & Alternative Medicine. Three of the physicians have worked alongside or on fellowship with the National Institute of Health or the National Institute on Drug Abuse. Four of the physicians teach or have taught medical school courses; eight have multiple peer-reviewed articles published within a defined medical specialty. Three have made notable contributions to medical cannabis research and one is in the final stages of publishing a book on Cannabis & Pain.

Only a few of the physicians (2 of 12) noted that they had very little experience recommending cannabis and "must see a few more patients before I get comfortable with the topic." More than half of the physician participants (8 of 12) operate or are involved with practices that specialize in Integrative Cannabis; four (4 of 12) work within hospital systems or private practice, including the two noted above who have only recently began making recommendations (Family Practice and Pain Specialty). Only three (3 of 12) physicians participating does not bill the service of "providing a medical cannabis recommendation" directly to the patient but includes it as a regular part of service that insurance plans normally cover as a regular office visit.

Four of the male physicians (4 of 10) acknowledged personal experience using cannabis for stress relief, spiritual awareness, and medical treatment. With one expressing,

"I stayed away from it for the most part. Until I finally didn't. When that happened, it was like well okay, this doesn't seem as dangerous as I was told. It can actually have some other benefits for anxiety. Wow!"

Another admitted that when he began working with cannabis patients: "I already had 50 years of experience using marijuana but mostly recreationally and spiritually. I used it pretty much on a weekly basis as part of my Sabbath ritual, but I had never had any experience using it medicinally." Only two physicians commented that they do not now nor have they "ever used cannabis for any reason."

The remaining six physicians (four male and two female) did not mention personal use. Yet, it appears, as one physician observes,

The medical profession and physicians are not unique [and their beliefs about cannabis use are] just a reflection of general society. I am sure that there are many of my peers who have used or are active users. Their opinions may be different than those of others. Some may think it is a dangerous drug or a drug full of other anecdotal negatives. I don't know how to quite say this, but it is just about drug use. It is the same thing as other recreational drugs that we know lead to serious health issues, like alcohol. And then, there is a certain moral component to it too. So, I think the medical community pretty well reflects the sentiments of society in general. I don't think it is as closed as people assume.

His reflection adequately demonstrates that it is the knowledge of cannabis research (including having pertinent information on the endocannabinoid system and the observational evidence presented by patients) that has played a key role in its medicinal acceptance by the physicians who participated in this study, and may in fact be beneficial for other physicians, policymakers, and patients to recognize. The integral approach also illuminates other challenges and issues affecting physicians by exposing the fundamental domains through which developmental change occurred for participants, as will be discussed in Chapter Four.

Patient Participants

20 registered cannabis patients participated in this study; 10 male and 10 female. As other studies consistently affirm medical cannabis patients are likely to be located, with lesser or greater degrees of social visibility, "all over the map" of actors and institutions (Hathaway et. al., 2011; Pedersen, 2009; Smucker Barnwell et. al., 2006, Earleywine, 2002) and this study's participants followed suit. The ages of participating patients ranged from 28 to 70. The majority (15 of 20) are Caucasian, the remaining five are of Hispanic or African American descent.

Of the patients participating in this study, five are permanently disabled due to illness or injury, 11 are working full-time jobs or are self-employed, four are working part-time jobs, including the one retired patient. Three (3 of 11) of the full-time employees are either U.S. federal employees or contractors and three (3 of 20) of the participants are veterans of the U.S. Military. All 20 operate or volunteer as medical cannabis advocates and have spoken publicly about his or her personal experiences as a medical cannabis patient. 15 of the patients participating in the study hold college degrees in a wide-range of disciplines and one is a licensed Naturopath. As noted, earlier, because the Naturopath is not a licensed M.D. or D.O. but is a registered cannabis patient, her responses were included within patient responses.

Each patient verified his or her medical cannabis patient status is currently valid and registered in one of the following medical cannabis states:

Washington (1)   California (3)   Colorado (6)

Arizona (2)   New Mexico (3)   Minnesota (1)

Illinois (3)   Connecticut (1)

More than half of participating patients (13 of 20) have relocated from another U.S. state to one of the ones listed above to access a medical cannabis program. U.S. States and territories patients have sought refuge from include:

Georgia (2)   Maryland (1)   Florida (2)

Missouri (1)   Oklahoma (2)   Texas (2)

Puerto Rico (1)   Mississippi (1)   South Carolina (1)

Discussion about these Medical Cannabis Refugees will continue in Chapter Five in relation to LR quadrant consequences.

Again, given that Mikuriya, et. al. (2007) found more than 95% of the patients were self-medicating prior to the receipt of a medical cannabis recommendation, it was not surprising to find that only two (2 of 20) of the patients received a medical cannabis recommendation from his or her primary or specialty physician. The remaining eighteen (18 of 20) utilized a medical cannabis evaluation center. Sixteen (16 of 18) specifically remarked that his or her "primary care doctor would not provide a medical cannabis recommendation," forcing them outside his or her normal health care system. Across the country this emerging medical cannabis evaluation system frequently forces patients to pay large sums for a recommendation from a physician they may or may not ever see again. Patients reported spending between $50 and $750 to satisfy the *bona-fide* doctor-patient relationship required by medical cannabis regulation in the U.S. states listed above in 2016.

In contrast with physicians, nearly every patient (19 of 20) cited previous experience using cannabis before they requested a medical cannabis recommendation. A medical cannabis refugee from Florida shares, "Before I relocated to become a patient, I began using cannabis in [home state]." Another patient from Colorado voices,

"I had been using marijuana for years, but didn't understand I was medicating and that I could be getting more benefit using it in other ways."

As mentioned in Chapter Two, physicians and patients are individual holons participating in roles (collective holons) within a greater holarchy that is the doctor-patient relationship and in the context, they are acting, such as a health care conversation about the recommendation of medical cannabis. The complexity of this relationship, as well as individual, cultural, or social values held about the context of the conversation, lends to the value of an AQAL frame.

By assessing the common and differing experiences of physicians and patients through an integral lens (Wilber, 2000a), while grounding the experiences in the solid AQAL theoretical frame, an authentic and interesting assessment of this phenomena emerged. This developed understanding of how doctors and patients communicate about the recommendation of medical cannabis will help guide future research, educational initiatives, and assist with normalizing the use of cannabis.

Interview Questions

In total, thirty-two (32) informed participants were asked open-ended questions regarding experiences related to the recommendation of medical cannabis. Probing questions, like the ones below, were asked if open-ended questions were not sufficient to accumulate applicable data:

1. Can you tell me how you came to recommend (physician) or request to be recommended (patient) medical cannabis?

   Physicians:

   a. Have you approached a patient about utilizing medical cannabis without the patient first requesting a recommendation? Describe a situation in which this occurred.

   b. How did you feel the first time a patient requested a medical cannabis recommendation from you? What concerns did this event bring up for you?

Patients:

    a. How did you come to medical cannabis as an option to consider in your own healthcare?

    b. How did you feel asking a doctor for a cannabis recommendation? What concerns did this event bring up for you?

2. Specific to the doctor-patient communication during the medical cannabis recommendation, can you describe your experiences recommending (physician) or receiving a recommendation (patient) for cannabis?

Physicians:

    a. In what ways does the conversation about medical cannabis differ from other conversations you engage in with patients?

    b. How do you feel about patients requesting a medical cannabis recommendation?

    c. How do you think these conversations are received by patients?

Patients:

    a. How did you feel about the consultation and your physician's response?

    b. What were your expectations prior to this conversation?

    c. Now that you're a registered patient, how do you communicate with physicians who provide care for you about your use of medical cannabis?

3. What did you learn from this experience? How does this affect you now?

Physicians:

    a. What tools or practices would help you with these conversations?

    b. What institutional or other concerns come into play during these conversations?

    c. What steps can be taken to improve the medical cannabis recommendation process?

Patients:

    a. What preparation, tools, or practices do you believe would have been helpful for you or your physician?

b. How has this experience affected your health care expectations, particularly the relationships you have with your physicians?

c. What steps can be taken to improve the medical cannabis recommendation process?

To help ensure validity, that participants were understood, and that any meaning interpreted was in fact a correct analysis, a follow-up with each participant occurred within ten (10) days after the initial interview was completed. All participants were asked to review the transcript from the interview for correctness and participants had an additional opportunity to contribute to the project with afterthoughts during the rough draft stage, as noted earlier. This data was combined with the transcripts to ensure clarity and understanding during data analysis.

In accordance with guidelines provided by Catherine Marshall and Gretchen Rossman (2011), following data collection, the raw narrative data from interviews were analyzed for "categories and themes" (p. 212) that were "clustered" or "sub-clustered" (p. 213) within the participant's narrative. The AQAL frame helped the researcher organize data into appropriate categories. "Salient themes, recurring ideas or language, and patterns of belief" (p. 214) that participants shared quickly became apparent. Narrative research dovetails with integral theory in that they all seek the truth of lived experience.

Adhering to the following steps guided the researcher during data analysis:

1. immersion in the transcripts
2. categorizing data into emerging themes and codes
3. coding the complete transcripts
4. creating an explanatory narrative that corresponds to the structure that emerged.

An integral understanding was developed from raw narrative data analysis on the subjective meaning to individual doctors and patients (UL); observations/demonstrations of individual behaviors shared narratively (UR); discussing tools and processes necessary on the collective level (LR), the uncovering of social and cultural characteristics that affect the conversation about medical cannabis recommendation (LR/LL), and developed an understanding of the relations between quadrants (AQAL) that affect the doctor-patient relationship. Narrative analysis allowed for view of these phenomena, as well as a view of the spaces in between, or the relation among the quadrants, as shared in Chapter Four.

Using Wilber's AQAL model, one can study the perspective of each quadrant from their complex interconnected relationships and as a holonic model, in that each quadrant is equally important to the whole. This project gathered narrative evidence to demonstrate the differences in the doctor's or patient's sense of self (UL), physical functioning and behaviors (UR), tools and processes used or needed (LL) and beliefs and values (LR). To increase the validity of the assessment, each narrative inquiry was transcribed and coded individually. Individual transcripts were independently coded prior to all physician interviews being comparatively analyzed, followed by patient interviews, and finally, a contrast of experiences of both participant groups was conducted. Data generated through audio transcripts, field notes, and collaboration with participants was categorized into the AQAL frame from the raw narratives to provide manageable data for investigation. As well, the AQAL framework was applied back to the data to illuminate the explanatory power contained within participant narrative.

Although health research (Baker and Watson, 2016; Gallois, 2009) has pointed to the problems in doctor–patient communication, it has not sufficiently investigated what patients or doctors think is happening during that communication or how these perceptions affect the doctor-patient relationship. Patients appreciate physicians who listen to them, allow them to ask questions, and who take the time to make sure they understand the patient's health condition and concerns. Positive engagement with a physician encourages patient communication, likewise a disorienting dilemma can shut communication down as this study demonstrates.

In Baker and Watson's (2016) recent study, "How Patients Perceive Their Doctors' Communication: Implications for Patient Willingness to Communicate," they conclude that,

"If health providers are aware of how patients interpret

physician behaviors, it may be possible to alter those behaviors in a way that favors patient participation in the consultation."

(p. 634). Since no published studies have examined the use of dialogic narratives as a knowledge tool for exploring and disseminating information gained from an analysis of the doctor-patient communication regarding medical cannabis recommendation, this study has an opportunity to positively impact doctor-patient communication from a broad perspective, by considering an issue that currently presents a disorienting dilemma to both parties.

Integral theory provides a meta-framework from which shared language, ideas, and concepts may be generated so a unified discourse may form. Applying this frame to the subject of medical cannabis recommendation opens the door for future research in many arenas.

Research Limitations

As cited in this study (Young, A., 2014; Ziemianski, D. et. al., 2015), there are several survey studies that begin to examine the complex issue of medical cannabis recommendation, but this study is among the first to take an in-depth examination of the issue of medical cannabis recommendation from the perspective of both parties involved in the process. Because this study chose a narrative format participants were asked to share personal perceptions so the data is subjective. The convenience sample limited the generalizability of the findings, since participants were not randomly selected.

As well, researcher familiarity had some impact with participants and may have affected how they responded. It is helpful to remember that while narrative inquiry is rich and substantive, it does not always produce conclusions of certainty, but rather focuses on the exploration and elaboration of complex human-centered processes (Clandinin, 2013).

This study was designed as an entry point to examining the issue of medical cannabis recommendation in more depth. These limitations point toward many complex areas of study that must be examined further, meeting the intent of the project.

Chapter Four

Research Findings

As discussed in Chapter Two, the AQAL (all-quadrants, all-levels) is a model and the foundational structure of *integral theory*; a method of integral methodological pluralism (IMP) that attempts to integrate as many valid systems of knowledge as possible into an inclusive, metatheoretical framework (Esbjorn-Hargens, 2009). AQAL has two axes: *the horizontal axis* denotes a continuum between interior and exterior realities and *the vertical axis* signifies a continuum between individual and collective realities. Together, the four quadrants represent the fundamental domains in which change and development occur in individuals and collective groups.

Using narrative data from one-on-one interviews with each study participant, the researcher explored the transcripts of individual stories, to discover the ways, in which participants had personally experienced the medical cannabis recommendation process, with all its complexities and critical events. How are doctors and patients - as participants in compassionate care programs - experiencing the medical cannabis recommendation process? From an AQAL perspective what are participant experiences telling us? And, are participants undergoing transformative learning as a result of these experiences?

The federal Controlled Substances Act (CSA), contributes to the complexity of the situation, as discussed in Chapter One. In this chapter, the narrative findings will be explored following the AQAL frame from the LR quadrant, where the CSA stems, to the LL quadrant, societal and cultural impacts from the CSA, to the UR quadrant, for a close view of the doctor-patient relationship, to the UL to consider interior themes from the personal perspective of participants. This chapter will conclude with an exploration into transformative learning trends discovered within the narrative data.

The communication between physicians and patients related to a medical cannabis recommendation is "perplexing for a wide-variety of reasons." Understanding the perspectives of both parties, from participants who have already successfully - and sometimes not so successfully - engaged in these conversations, is a vital place to begin. How does requesting or offering a medical cannabis recommendation affect (AQAL) the participant's: doctor and patient? What are the factors they consider?

The following themes were unearthed early in the data collection process:

1. The federal CSA has a trickledown effect in the LR quadrant to State Public Health Institutions and local medical institution policy. The cumulative effect marginalizes and affects decision-making for system participants across AQAL.

2. Society, and therefore, communities and cultures are transitioning to new social constructs about what it means to use cannabis (LL) and to be a cannabis user (UL). At this critical juncture, public and professional education and social support are necessary, for participants in medical cannabis systems and communities.

3. The doctor-patient relationship is directly and negatively impacted by the CSA, and the LR debris it causes. A frequent and costly side-effect is fragmentation of patient care and disruption of doctor-patient relations (UR).

4. Cultural perceptions (LL) about alternative health care, Holistic Medicine, and substance abuse and addiction seep heavily into myths and taboos about cannabis use.

5. Physicians and patients have both experienced internalized fear, loss of status, stigmatizing judgment, and have been denied personal expression (UL) because of the continued prohibition of cannabis the CSA reinforces.

6. Transformative learning experiences are common within the medical cannabis community, as observed and exhibited in participant stories.

LR: Institutions, Systems, and Processes

The following section explores the LR or Exterior Collective quadrant representing the collective perspectives as addressed by this study's thirty-two (32) patient and physician participants. Given the Schedule I status of cannabis, the CSA figures prominently into participant narrative. This Arizona patient's story illuminates the harsh realities the LR quadrant inflicts on AQAL:

> *The plant is not doing them harm, but the laws and the people who are profiting from the prohibition are the ones who are caught in the harm. Among those I include not just the police, but courts, lawyers, drug-testing, the black market itself benefits tremendously, even international cartels who illegally bring drugs into the country benefit...the prison complex, N.I.D.A., the D.E.A. particularly, and all the other benefactors... All of these ills come from prohibition, not cannabis itself. When I see this drug that is helpful to me and so many other people being vilified, to put it lightly, I feel a very strong desire to stand up to that. To try to affect some kind of change to turn the situation around because it is not sustainable in the long-term...The sooner we can change to a sustainable national policy regarding cannabis, and other drugs as well, the better off we - as a society - will be. The War*

on Drugs is a war on our own people. It must stop!

The list of questions a physician must ask him or herself before making a medical cannabis recommendation for an inquiring patient is long and complex: "How will it impact my license? My ability to code and bill? Or do all the things that keep me afloat and practicing? Are they going to come after me? Is the D.E.A. going to come after me? Am I really allowed to sign that? Can I sign that? Am I protected or am I putting my license at risk?" Every physician (12 of 12) shared that the Schedule I status of cannabis "definitely has an effect here." The first question they each asked themselves was,

"Is this even *legal*?"

After having experience working with patients in this area, each listed *reclassification* (8 of 12; "Even a reschedule would be helpful for research and legal purposes"/"Rescheduling is necessary for medical acceptance and validity") or *declassification* (4 of 12; "Complete removal from the Controlled Drug Schedule is what science proves"/"It is a nutritional supplement, like a vitamin, it needs to be removed from the Schedule altogether") as the greatest impediment to acceptance within the medical community and the population-at-large. They also acknowledged it as the "greatest area of fear for those practicing" in this arena. One physician confirms,

> *We've got more and more states passing medical programs or*
> *decriminalization. The federal government should look at it*
> *again. The first step is to get it reclassified. It should easily go*
> *down the schedule or be removed. Either way that will allow*
> *some research - good research and human studies - to finally*
> *be done. N.I.D.A. needs to put more money towards that...*
> *There's good research in Europe, in the Middle East, and [other*
> *countries] - people around here aren't willing to look at it.*
> *There is good research but for some reason you've got*
> *physicians thinking if it didn't come from the United States, it*

ain't worth diddly. We need good research - period - for some of their eyes to open and to turn their heads around - so they'll be saying, 'Maybe there is something to this.' Get the government to change their stance - allow some good research to be done and then, we'll have more providers."

Another physician shares,

Research is coming, but it's been very slow because it's been illegal all these years. There has been no funding for studies. Doctors usually don't change their mind about anything until there are studies that demonstrate the effectiveness of a new drug, or a new therapeutic modality, or anything. Very often, if there is just one study, then that's not enough either. They need multiple studies demonstrating the same thing. We tend to be a highly critical group.

Unfortunately, now, "Three generations have grown up believing that there is something terribly wrong and harmful with marijuana and that getting high was dangerous!" and

"Three generations of doctors have learned the wrong information about this medicine."

The Schedule I status is a very difficult hurdle for most physicians and institutions to overcome, because it "incorrectly classifies marijuana as having no medicinal value. And it certainly does!"

When a patient considers registering as a medical cannabis patient within his or her state's medical cannabis program, the list of questions they must ask themselves is also long and complex. It also begins with, "Is this even legal?" As well, they must be able and prepared to undertake a great deal of paperwork and willing to risk social stigma (LL), as this study finds. For all twenty (20 of 20) patients participating in this study, the sentiment is virtually the same as this patient, "The prohibition that is prescribed to deal with the *supposed* menace is actually causing *all* the harm."

Patients also gave reference to other systemic issues driven by the Schedule I status of *cannabis sativa*. Several commented on the inherent nature of the CSA status to discriminate. "This schedule was put in place to control people: brown and black people." "In this system, there is room for systemic racism. There's room for discrimination. There's room for preferences. It is systemic racism." Primarily, patients shared "disbelief" regarding the U.S. government's failure to reclassify cannabis.

"The way the federal government has put together this Schedule doesn't help. I mean, cannabis scheduled along with heroin? Really?"

Though only two physicians (2 of 12 or 16%) mentioned PubMed as a good resource for cannabinoid research, fourteen (14 of 20 or 70%) of the patients noted this resource by name, as they shared personal stories. Patients noted that "credible online sources" had helped them locate "factual" information, including "many clinical and animal studies." The safety profile, "cannabis is non-toxic," (32 of 32 participants) is the primary reason each participant, physician or patient, believed it should be rescheduled, if not completely descheduled. "De-schedule, not reschedule." Eighteen (18 of 20) patient participants mentioned, "personal research" led them to believe "science supports de-scheduling" cannabis.

Additionally, twelve (12 of 20) patients discussed "cannabis as food" as reasoning for it to be removed from the List of Controlled Substances. "We've got to be looking at medicine from a level of nutrition. Cannabis is food on a cellular level. It provides cellular nutrition." Finally, "I just pray they [D.E.A.] will de-schedule" were words that were repeated verbatim by four patients, in three separate states, who've never met. This type of passion expresses the frustration between a Schedule I status (LR) and a patient's embodied knowledge (UL), cultural (LL), and relational (UR) experiences.

Political Power-as-Dominance:
D.E.A. Interference

The tangled web of public policies, state regulations, and institutional policies and practices are LR challenges with AQAL effects, that both parties face given the Schedule I status of *cannabis sativa*. Patient participants (13 of 20) also recognize the fear doctors have about risking a medical license or D.E.A. prescription capabilities. "Why is her license at risk if she helps me live longer and feel better? I really do not understand how law enforcement has this much authority over medical decisions."

Physician participants (12 of 12) share beliefs that "things won't change significantly until the Schedule I status changes." As well, they acknowledge (12 of 12) that hospital and clinic systems in the U.S. are connected tightly with - and reliant upon - federal funding, "which may be put at risk" if the institution becomes involved with a Schedule I drug. "It is still federally illegal. Those laws still have not changed; meaning any facility that takes federal funds, which is a lot with Medicaid and Medicare." Institutions are at risk of losing federal funding.

Physicians are also registered and tracked by the D.E.A. regarding all Schedule drug prescribing habits. Cannabis lies outside this system, since it can only be recommended not prescribed, but that doesn't stop the D.E.A from intimidating physicians as a Colorado physician affirms,

> There's a fear among doctors that they'll lose their D.E.A. registration. The D.E.A. just doesn't want physicians to recommend marijuana and prescribe opiates at the same time ...Patients [regularly ask] 'Can you prescribe my pain pills?' I say, "No, I am just focusing on the marijuana, that's enough." I don't even want to mix it because, you know, that the Feds, the D.E.A., are always watching.

Another conveys,

> A lot of doctors are apprehensive about participating in the medical cannabis program. They are afraid they will get

raided and the state licensing bureau is going to come down on
them. It's unwarranted, but there is still a real palpable fear
among practicing physicians.

Nearly every Integrative Cannabis physician that participated in this study (9 of 12) discussed his or her concern of "the D.E.A. policing my medical practice." The only four (4 of 12) physicians not discussing this concern work under the umbrella of a large hospital or clinic system and "are subject to much less risk there."

Most of the Integrative Cannabis physicians (5 of 8) voice examples of D.E.A. agents threatening them; none of the private or hospital affiliated physicians (4 of 12) disclosed a similar experience. A physician in California relays,

They asked if I was writing opiate prescriptions. Once I told
them I don't; that instead I help people wean off the opiates
and narcotics, they left and I went back to work.

A physician in Colorado describes his experience,

It's unsettling for patients to see D.E.A. jacket-wearing officers
waiting in my office and it is frustrating for me because I abide
by all laws. To me, it is just a form of harassment that is
uncalled for in this day and age.

Another physician describes the D.E.A. interference in medical decisions via threats to suspend a doctor's D.E.A. prescribing rights, as he has experienced it,

The challenge for some of my patients is that a great deal of the
clinics and the physicians around here pull this number on
them: They say, 'Well I can't prescribe you opiates when you're
using marijuana because that's against the law.' I say, 'Ask
them for proof of that law.' Of course, there is no such law.
There is no law that says you can't use or prescribe opiates and
cannabis together. If there was I couldn't do it. And I do it!
There is no state or federal law that says you can't...I've even

*talked with D.E.A. Officers in my office. They know exactly
what I'm doing and I've been doing it for a long time. It's just
amazing what the rest of the medical community will do, in my
opinion. Unethically lie to patients by saying, 'I can't do that, it
is illegal.' They just don't want to do it. They are letting their
own biases and prejudices get in the way of treatment.*

Perhaps, fear of "losing one's practice" or "having to deal with the harassment" are also contributing factors. In each state that has medicalized cannabis use, D.E.A. agents "regularly meet with cannabis doctors," an act that can be defined as "aggressive" and "intimidating" by some (7 of 12). As a Nevada physician shares,

*Two D.E.A. agents came to my office three weeks after I signed
a recommendation for the first time. They flat out told me I
could prescribe opiates or cannabis, but I can't prescribe both.*

He went on to share,

*How is it they have a voice in a medical decision between a
patient and me? They're not doctors! They don't even
acknowledge it has medical value - and, that's why.*

Most physicians shared stories of these visits. Typically, these visits in the doctor's office, are in front of patients and staff. "Usually during the busiest part of the day so they have to sit and wait among patients." D.E.A. "jackets and guns holstered" for effect, described by one doctor as,

*An intimidation tactic that works better on the patient than the
physician. I've had patients decide they didn't want to get
certified after encountering that display in a doctor's office.
I've had staff quit because they were afraid. But, this doctor -
she stays! I've seen too many medical miracles to give up now.
I had no idea I had this kind of fight left in me!*

71

Each of the physicians that participated in the study (12 of 12) self-educated about the legal ramifications of recommending cannabis before engaging in the practice. Though D.E.A. interference often still occurred at some point in the Integrative Cannabis practices it was described by several physicians as "less legally concerning than just a bullying threat from the feds."

While it would seem safe for a physician to provide a medical cannabis recommendation given the above information, three (3 of 20) patients in three states (Colorado, New Mexico, and Minnesota) reported that shortly after a first recommendation was approved by a physician, either his or her license was suspended or charges of inappropriate prescription writing were brought against the doctor in question. A Colorado patient claims, "I walked out of my recommendation appointment to find two D.E.A. agents sitting in the lobby. I just about fainted. That's really intimidating!" A Minnesota patient shares, "Three days after I was certified, the doctor was arrested for 33 counts of prescription fraud or something. It scared me. I mean I was just forced to see a doctor who may be acting fraudulently. Wow!"

A New Mexico patient shares,

> Three local pain specialists, who were certifying patients after much convincing, got their licenses taken and were sued for malpractice for over-prescribing opiates, defrauding Medicare. Suddenly, there were no pain specialists available. We had to send patients to another city - four hours away. This was another financial hardship for patients. It's been rough, very rough for the pain patients. And, I know because I am one of them.

Actions like these by D.E.A. chapters across the country send shock waves and fear, though not only the local medical community, but the local medical cannabis patient community in each instance. Chapter Five's section on Additional Findings suggests further research into the Schedule I status and its extra-legal consequences is warranted. The findings below are directly tied to the federal CSA's prohibition of *cannabis sativa.*

Knowledge Control: Research Hindered

Schedule I status has had an enormously negative impact on research. In effect, it prohibits the medical establishment's preferred model, the randomized clinical trial (RCT), as mentioned in Chapter One. The extended prohibition of cannabis has also had an enormously negative impact on our understanding of the endocannabinoid system (eCS) and the phytocannabinoids of the *cannabis sativa* plant, hindering scientific and medical knowledge. Though much exists, far more remains "a distant hope, for the most part." Schedule I status restricts clinical research, much less any attempt at disseminating a public health message. "Cannabis is on the Schedule I list. Doctors can't even look at cannabis like it has any kind of medical value because of that." Funding is simply not allocated for projects that consider the medical efficacy of a Schedule I substance in humans. An Integrative Cannabis physician interested in conducting medical cannabis human trials asserts,

> *Unless you are studying its adverse effects; you can't get any funds to study cannabis at all. No institution wants to be studying its medicinal benefit. It is still a Schedule I drug. It can't have medical validity before the government says it does. We have enough good research to prove that true already. Cannabis has a ton of medical validity and many applications but until the government says 'Go!' by changing the Schedule or removing it, as they should, institutions are not going to challenge it.*

A Washington physician shared how this LR division affects his relationship (UL) with patients,

> *Some of this is obviously the federal intransigent and shows how dependent we are on our system of state and federal in harmony with health care. Hopefully, that will change soon but in the meantime, the states really do need to step up. States with medical marijuana programs should be investing in*

research and educating physicians and the public about its
safety and benefits.

Though LR policy is to blame, this physician, like others, has been stigmatized within his profession (LL), as well as individually (UL), as a result. Further, neither physicians nor patients can fully answer the question "Will this work for me?" or "Will this work for my patient?"- which is another important decision factor for both parties in a medical cannabis recommendation conversation. The CSA status impedes research and the dissemination of information that can help both parties begin to answer these and other questions of importance.

While the body of government and publicly funded cannabinoid research is slim, patients appear to have even less patience with the federal restrictions than do physicians. One Colorado patient shares,

> *We're just not going to do it? We are just going to leave people*
> *to suffer until we get the research doctors desire? I support the*
> *research, but I don't want patients to have to suffer until the*
> *medical community gets everything it wants. All the*
> *information they want is years down the road. In the*
> *meantime, patients are suffering and dying.*

Another Colorado patient states,

> *Doctors educate themselves for years and years on their*
> *specialty or their practice. Cannabis is just not part of it. It's*
> *like a new disease that's just been discovered, except it is a new*
> *system of the body. People are researching it to figure out what*
> *it is and what to do with it. But, it doesn't correlate with me*
> *that we don't know enough. There are plenty of scientific*
> *studies out there if you just take the time to read them.*

Other patients reaffirmed the stories of physicians, as well as explain the potentially stigmatizing outcome of having too few RCTs to meet the needs of doctors. An Illinois patient conveys,

When I told him, "I've seen research studies on this," he said, "Well, it isn't proven." He just shut me off. It wasn't even something he'd consider discussing with me.

Given how much information is available online through reputable academic sources, patients (20 of 20) have the "expectation of my doctors that they know about the endocannabinoid system."

"It's a shame that there are no pharmaceutical reps telling them about [Cannabis]. They'd be amazed if they heard that news from the government or the National Institutes of Health."

Given the D.E.A. interference, both physicians and patients are resigned that until the Schedule I status changes, "There aren't going to be any human studies done. We can't do those now because of the Schedule I status."

State Compassionate Care Policies

While sharing stories, participating patients (20 of 20) also share the importance of traversing his or her state's medical cannabis system and being "acknowledged as a medical cannabis patient." An Illinois patient proudly reflected on receiving his medical cannabis card, "I actually got it - I will never forget the day! November 6th, 2015 at 2:30pm. But, then the dispensaries weren't even open." Every patient shared "excitement" to the effect, "I will never forget the day I received my patient card. I had so much hope after trudging down such a long, hard path."

Several *medical cannabis refugees*, as will be discussed, voice "I moved my family halfway across the country for this little card right here. Was it worth it? Yes! Yes! Yes! I am living proof it was worth it!" Another, who relocated from Puerto Rico to the U.S. mainland for cannabis therapy, said this about receiving his first medical cannabis recommendation,

It gives me freedom to be a patient. It legitimized the causes and it legitimized my use. Back in the day, I was feeling oppressed. I felt like an outlaw because I was consuming this plant illegally. I was constantly hiding. I was living a double-life with self-medication.

Patients who have registered as cannabis patients "believed this program would benefit me, but found it more difficult to get registered than I ever thought possible." The two primary reasons for difficulty were "finding a doctor who would do the recommendation" and "dealing with the registration process through the Public Health Department." As relayed through participant stories, public health departments influence a participant's decision-making, whether the individual decides to join the system or not.

Public Health Departments

From a policy and regulation perspective, navigating a Health Department's medical cannabis program's application and registry process - as well as obtaining a recommendation from a physician - are the first courses of action and sometimes the most difficult feats to achieve for patients. These actions often occur months before the elusive medical cannabis card arrives and only "after extensive research." Since, physician participants admitted that patients frequently lead the conversation about medical cannabis recommendation and patient testimonial confirms that most start by researching the program requirements, consideration must be given to experiences with the programs administered by any State's Department of Health. The experience with the Department of Health affects decision-making regarding the recommendation of medical cannabis. The experience can be discouraging for potential patients or physicians. As one New Mexico patient describes Health Departments "aren't renowned for good communication."

It was more than two years after the vote that we finally

started learning about the program. The Health Department was very slow, often very confusing, and obviously not patient-centered in its approach to medical marijuana.

A Colorado patient affirms,

You could get your medical marijuana license before I knew, of course. It had been enacted into law, but they'd kept it kind of quiet, squashed it. The information wasn't out there.

An Arizona patient shares this type of experience is challenging for many patients,

It was a difficult and unnecessarily cumbersome process that would be particularly difficult for people without computer skills, internet access, or adequate time to figure out what to do.

An Illinois patient's story encapsulates the responses of several other patients in regards to support received from a State Department of Public Health,

It's like they don't want anyone to register for the program, if they did it wouldn't be so difficult. Terminally and chronically ill people are the only ones eligible, yet the process is so difficult, I've already known three patients to die before they got their card. That isn't right or what the voters of this state wanted.

Predominantly, patients conveyed that,

"[My] medical cannabis program is not what the voters of this state wanted when the initiative passed, but it's what we got, so we try our best to deal with it."

Participating patients (12 of 12) find medical cannabis programs to be marginalizing and difficult to navigate, particularly as a new program emerges. Unfortunately, over time "the problems, not only don't get better, new problems - systemic, bureaucratic problems - come up." One Oregon physician states,

> *The Department of Health is no help. They don't even know how their own rules and regulations will work until they roll them out. Then they see how badly they've hurt us. However, they seldom change to something better, they just keep hurting us.*

A California physician shares how medical cannabis programs differ from other support he receives,

> *Any state that passes a medical cannabis law should be required to educate physicians through their local Health Department. These agencies already run physician education programs, this is just one more - but, it actually has funding behind it to pay for the education. We don't have to deal with them much here, but then again we don't get any support from them either.*

Physicians do not have a better relationship than patients with the State Department of Health based on participant input. "The Department of Health is the culprit. They are taking forever to certify or recertify patients." One New Mexico patient, a naturopath, comments on the social harm patients she's encountered have experienced based on the federal Schedule I status of cannabis.

> *When a patient on probation's medical card expires and his urine tests positive for THC, well, he goes to jail. This happens a lot because the Health Department takes so long to recertify patients.*

The delays for certification or recertification in New Mexico have been made public (Teague, 2016). A New Mexico physician also expressed concerns about these delays,

> *I recertified patients for renewals more than four months ago. Those patients have gone at least a month, some two, without access to medication simply because the Department of Health is running behind.*

Doctor and patient participants (30 of 32) coalesced on the fact that "Anytime you deal with any kind of state paperwork, it is intimidating" and both parties believe,

"There needs to be a strategic plan put into place about how this is going to be regulated and how people are going to be educated and informed about it."

For physician participants (10 of 12) dealing with the recommendation paperwork is often "unnecessarily confusing and time consuming." Trying to figure out "how to stay on the straight and narrow with very unclear definitions from the state" is also frustrating. An Arizona physician insists,

> *I am very careful to make sure that whatever we submit is compatible with the state guidelines...then you add the implied and sometimes not implied threat to physicians, who are trying to practice medicine. It's a real palpable fear with practicing physicians.*

Like this Oregon physician, participating doctors (12 of 12) are frustrated by the lack of support they've received from State Health Departments.

> *The State's Health Department provides my staff and me information on every new flu season's vaccine, HIV/AIDS updates, senior health issues, prenatal health issues, etcetera.*

But, they were not able to give me any information on how patients are using cannabis? I had to find that out by asking patients. Once I asked enough patients...I thought, I knew more than the Health Department about it, so I took them information for other physicians. That was two years ago, I give them an updated version twice a year because I am learning so much. They've yet to share it with any other doctors. My patients though, they share it with all of their other doctors. Their other doctors have now started referring more patients to me because they'd rather they be seen by someone who knows about cannabis, tracks the patient, and provides good care, than to see them go to these evaluation mills that are popping up everywhere.

An Arizona physician affirms,

The rules and regulations aren't complicated once you've spent hours understanding what it is that the state requires. It would be helpful to have the health department provide that for all physicians or healthcare networks in the state. If they did, a few institutions might still prohibit recommendations but not the majority. Also, physicians might provide recommendations as a normal part of patient care. These healthcare mega-conglomerates that often operate as NPOs don't really seem to want to support patients or their own programs in that way.

He went on to share, "They also don't want to risk their federal funding." Of course, they don't.

Insurance Companies

The health insurance coverage of patients excludes medical cannabis evaluation, unless covered as "a regular part of a normal office visit." It also excludes cannabis medication. Each physician (12 of 12) commented on how this obstacle affects patients.

"Nothing is covered by insurance...that's hard on patients."

Doctors recognize and patient testimony confirms, medical cannabis can quickly become an "unaffordable process and medication" for patients seeking care outside normal healthcare systems. "You don't get reimbursement for medical cannabis, at all. And, certainly not for the medication. That's very inhibiting for a lot of people." An Illinois physician specializing in pain management shares,

> A great deal of pain is stress and anxiety induced: the patient gets injured: finances become a problem, family life, the marriage, everything starts to become a big issue.

A Colorado physician affirms,

> Now that cannabis is truly their only medicine in many cases, not having coverage can become a burdensome expense for disabled patients and the families of disabled children who've come to Colorado for cannabis therapy.

For doctors, insurance extends beyond the companies they rely on and deal with for patient benefits and service payments to medical malpractice and other business liability requirements they must meet to practice medicine. Each insurance organization establishes independent policies and practices (LR), meaning it is often difficult for doctors to find support should they decide to work with medical cannabis patients and submit medical cannabis recommendations to the state. Insurance company guidelines are strict LR influences on policies and practices, because the "financial rewards aren't worth risking."

For physician participants, another major obstacle to overcome is the requirement for malpractice insurance and other business insurances medical practices rely upon. As a Colorado physician shares,

> "The medical malpractice insurance companies, early on said, 'Don't be writing these' or they put limits on it. You can only do a certain number."

While sharing her story, she also states,

> *It was a whole thing where the insurance companies sent out letters saying, 'If you do this, we're going to drop you - we're not insuring it - not only are we not insuring you for those activities, we will drop you!' so that's the big chill...Now, I do have a personal malpractice insurance that's required in the state for financial responsibility. I have a special policy that covers the medical marijuana evaluation, but I am not covered for anything else. So, there is this divide.*

Institutional Policies

The above concerns tie to the CSA and the resulting institutional policies that prohibit associated physicians from recommending cannabis are still quite common. In fact, these policies help support the medical cannabis evaluation clinic model as it is the best available option for most patients. It also offers a relatively "stigma-free recommendation experience" for most, as this study's participants affirm (17 of 20). A Colorado patient shares,

> *I went to the clinic to see my regular doctor first. I asked if she could write the recommendation for me. Fortunately, the doctor was very open and quite pro-cannabis and I understood she wasn't against it, but she couldn't write the recommendation*

because the clinic she works for is federally-funded. They all are, I think.

An Arizona patient imparted a similar story,

> *He was a doctor at the University Medical Center. I asked him about a recommendation. He said he'd been told by the Board of Directors that their doctors would not be allowed to do them. Period.*

This situation forces patients to pay not only out-of-pocket for medical cannabis products, but to find and cash pay a physician for a recommendation as well. Another Colorado patient, shares her story,

> *My prescriptions are paid for by my insurance company but my insurance will not pay for my medical marijuana card, the doctor's visit to get the recommendation, or the medicine I buy that actually helps my spasticity and my pain…Every single year, I must come up with $200 for a doctor renewal. Then every month I must come up with money for my medicine. My insurance has saved a ton of money. They have saved money on doctor visits, hospital visits, Emergency Room visits, and prescriptions because I began using cannabis.*

Cost is always a factor of consideration and when insurance won't cover an expense, like the recommendation for medical cannabis itself, a patient must consider the LR consequences against UL benefits. As one small business owner and Illinois patient shares,

> *Of course, the insurance wasn't going to cover it. I had to pay out-of-pocket for all of that; the doctor's visits, the background check, the fingerprints. Insurance wasn't going to cover all that and I didn't expect they would. To me, I rationalized it. The cost was this against the long-term side-effects of the medications*

83

they had me taking. I'm a small business owner, I could
rationalize the cost upfront because in the long run it is going
to help save my organs.

For pain patients and physicians, who specialize in pain management, the drug testing policy many institutions mandate is one of the most difficult obstacles to overcome. For patients, it often means changing physicians or sometimes even medical systems. For doctors, it becomes a push against the larger institution, but as one describes, it's an issue of importance,

Our patient population is coming in for opiates and narcotics
and testing positive for all this marijuana. We had to quit
testing for the marijuana or we would have had to fire
probably 50% or more of the patients in our practice. They
were all using it illegally... We have 17,000 patients. We had to
quit testing for THC so that we could - we would -
stop firing these patients. Because it is an illicit drug and if you
have an illicit drug in your system and we have it in the policy
that you can't, you've got to change that policy.

Though several participants, both patients and physicians note that pain management policies are changing, these changes often come "too slowly for patient relief."

In fact, medical institutions are renown for zero tolerance drug policies meaning that pre-employment, random (in some cases), and workman's compensation-related injuries will expose the employee to drug testing that includes THC. For this reason, it was unexpected to have a full third of physician participants (4 of 12) share personal experiences using cannabis. As well, five (5 of 12) physicians remarked about zero tolerance drug policies, but only discussed the negative effects on patients. A Connecticut physician conveys,

I've had two patients denied employment because they are
medical marijuana patients. If I gave them Marinol they'd

pass, but because they use the plant they fail. This doesn't seem right.

An Illinois Pain Specialist frustratingly shares,

I have a patient and I thought the medical cannabis would be a good option for her. Then she goes to get a job, applies for the job, and they urine test her. She tests positive for THC because she's on the medical marijuana program. They said, 'Sorry we can't hire you.' That needs to be changed!

Zero tolerance drug policies frequently extend to social service policies, as another physician shares,

Child Protective Services was trying to take a mother's custody away based on the fact she has THC in her system. She's a registered marijuana patient. Of course, she will have THC in her system. Why are they even testing for it if she's allowed it? It is far better than her being on opiates!

Nearly half of the patient participants (8 of 20) also remarked about drug testing in the workplace, including a U.S. veteran who had been discharged from military service due to cannabis use "I tested positive for THC in 2001, but was positively discharged because I was honest and came forward with my cannabis use." Several (5 of 20) revealed that employment-related drug testing was a primary concern they'd had prior to requesting a medical cannabis recommendation. Loss of employment, loss of status with current or prospective employers were significant factors in patient decision-making for four others (4 of 20).

"Once you're a legal cannabis consumer, you are out of bounds for many legal actions, but

there are barriers to getting employment."

Another's story of recovery has her internalizing fear (UL) about her return to the workforce,

> Now as I am seeking employment, a drug test might become an issue. I might have to disclose to an employer that I am a medical cannabis patient. I am concerned this might be another thing to overcome as I am trying to get back into the workforce.

As the participants recognize and share, "Patients are extremely vulnerable in the system. Oftentimes, they are very disempowered."

Medical Cannabis Evaluation Centers: A Fragmentation of Healthcare

A few participating patients (5 of 20) said,

"I've just chosen to go to an evaluation center instead of my own doctor just to keep the two separate. I don't want any repercussions, whether it is in terms of health care coverage or legal liability or anything else."

Each of these patients researched the options and "felt that going to an evaluation center and never mentioning it to my doctor was the best option for me, at that time." However, most (15 of 20) have asked a primary or specialty physician for a recommendation or a renewal (registrations must be updated at least annually in all medicalized states). "Why should I have to deal with that from my doctors? It is easier this way...It's not so awkward." In every case (15 of 20), the patient was denied a recommendation and "felt forced to go to a marijuana doctor," outside his or her normal healthcare and insurance systems. There is still a stigma associated with this, even though more than half of the U.S. has medicalized cannabis programs.

How do doctors feel about patients getting pushed out of the regular medical systems? Most, including all of those who have established an Integrative Cannabis practice (9 of 12) voice, "I don't feel good about it. I think it leads to the fragmentation of health care." Those with Integrative Cannabis practices have little worry about attracting patients, few even advertise. A Colorado physician shares,

> *Patients share my information with others. It's all word of*
> *mouth. Our clinic is scheduled for three months in advance.*

However, "if you haven't got regulatory support from your system" or "you get pushed outside normal healthcare systems" supporting patients in this way may not be advantageous to your long-term career. Another Colorado physician shares, "I have been denied several promotions through my hospital system because I've started doing recommendations against policy. But, seeing my patients wean opiates and narcotics makes the battle and the disrespect worth it."

From a patient's (20 of 20) perspective, medical cannabis evaluation centers are "expensive and completely unnecessary." "It's an unnecessary restriction." "If you must buy and manage your own medicine, then why do I have to scramble to find a doctor? He's not helping me anyway." As well, most experience that, "It is disjointed. We have our cannabis care and we have our medical care; the two don't have any association." Further, there are "a lot of fly-by-night" medical cannabis evaluation centers. Four of the patient participants (4 of 20) share experiences with this area of concern. "These places pop up, make a ton of money in a few months, usually the last 100 or so patients are denied by the state because the group wasn't meeting the requirements to recommend."

> *Medical groups that advertise on social media are the worst.*
> *They may be real doctors but they only care about real money.*
> *They have no helpful advice and I don't want to be caught*
> *using a scam doctor.*

In an Illinois patient's story, we can see how uncomfortable some of the evaluation center experiences are for patients.

> *They gave me a referral to a doctor. I went to go see this guy. It was in this little office way up high in a little building. It took 45 minutes and was creepy, bizarre, or something. He just sat there and stared at me for a long time. "When you take cannabis how does it make you feel?" Makes me feel better than when I don't use it? I didn't know how to answer most of his questions, they just seemed weird or he made me feel weird. He started writing a lot of things down suddenly and I didn't know what he was going to do. But, he did write my recommendation. I won't use him again though. I have trouble understanding why my own doctor can't support this since he knows the success I'm having with it.*

Further insights about how participants experience this fragmentation will be included in the UR quadrant discussion and in Chapter Five.

Patient Rights

Patient rights were mentioned by ten (10 of 12) doctors participating in this study. The two main areas of focus for physicians were 1) medical records and 2) drug testing by pain management clinics. Additionally, eighteen (18 of 20) patients mentioned patient rights in the two areas noted by physicians, as well as discussing "healthcare and social providers not understanding I have rights as a medical marijuana patient." As both parties acknowledged during interviews, patients often do not know the rights they have associated with healthcare information, including access to medical records. More specifically, patients frequently do not know the content of personal medical records. Several participant physicians are "appalled by the content of some of the patient's records." An Oregon physician elucidates,

> *I get records from everybody. Most of the marijuana clinics*

around here, say, "Oh, come in with your last two visits from
your doctor and we'll get you approved." They don't
look at those records. They look and it says pain,
so you're qualified. For a brand-new patient, I require the last
two full years of every single medical provider they have seen
including urgent care and E.R. I personally review all that to
get a big picture of this person. I have no problem
showing them their own medical records: what is says,
what has been documented, what has not been documented,
what other doctors failed to see, and important labs or other
information. Sometimes they are astounded.

Another physician suggests,

More patients need to read their own medical records. They ne
ed to get more involved with their own health care. They leave
it to the doctor thinking the doctor has got their best interest
in mind. That's not always true. Because the doctor is so busy
sometimes, he can make mistakes. He could fail to see
something. They need to stay on top of them to make sure
they're getting these things done right.

Of the 20 patient participants, 13 mention gaining access to medical records as "stressful" or they had found "it difficult and because of hospital policies it took a very long time to get all my records together." A patient that now volunteers helping others register as a medical cannabis patient shares,

Even just asking for their patient records is hard for some
patients. They really have a hard time; just having the
conversation about requesting records with just the nurse or
administrative staff...People don't even know their own rights
to their own medical history. This is a source of anxiety
because they feel that they're asking for something that maybe

isn't even theirs to have.

A surprising number of participating patients (7 of 20) shared that "marijuana addict or marijuana abuse" (UL/LL) had been noted in medical records by a physician (6 male, 1 female). This note was from a primary or specialty physician they'd asked about a medical cannabis recommendation. One cancer-survivor was shown that his records reflected "marijuana abuse" by an Integrative Cannabis physician in Illinois.

> *Marijuana abuser? Really, I hadn't used cannabis in 18 years*
> *at the time I asked for a medical cannabis recommendation.*
> *But, I'm glad I pursued it and that the medical cannabis doctor*
> *told me about that being in my record. I went to the doctor and*
> *confronted him. He said he would remove it from my records.*
> *I've never abused anything!*

A U.S. military veteran who relocated from Georgia to Colorado in 2014 to try cannabis therapy in a desperate attempt to save his own life shares a frustration from this journey.

> *I've been a cannabis patient for three years. I began talking to*
> *my V.A. doctors about using cannabis after I became a legal*
> *patient. My medical records now reflect that I am a chronic*
> *marijuana abuser as a diagnosis. How ridiculous is that? I*
> *counted, they prescribed me 42 different prescriptions over the*
> *five years prior to my becoming a cannabis patient. None of*
> *those worked! I try something that works for my pain and my*
> *P.T.S. and they say I am a chronic abuser? It's ludicrous!*

In total, seven patient participants (7 of 20) noted they had been labeled (LL/UL) a "chronic marijuana abuser" or "marijuana addict" by a primary or specialty physician, but were "unaware that had been done until the marijuana doctor showed me my records."

In regard to this inappropriate labeling of a patient, participating physicians (5 of 12) testimony substantiated these concerns. An Oregon physician shares that,

"Marijuana abuser appears in patient records pretty frequently - placed there by uneducated and uncaring physicians, as approved by the administration. It really is horrifying."

The participants who are federal contractors (3 of 20) and veterans (3 of 20) shared UL internalized fears about this type of scenario or had already experienced it (6 of 20).

Medical vs. Recreational Cannabis Use

Though the medicalization of cannabis is quite different than policies in Colorado, Washington, Oregon, and others which are emerging (California, Maine, Massachusetts, and Nevada) that decriminalize adult use of cannabis, both types of policy violate the federal CSA. Physicians practicing within these three states (5 of 12) have "noticed a considerable change in attitude" among his or her peers and medical institutions based upon the state's 'legalization' initiatives. Now that any adult over the age of 21 has legal access to cannabis, patients are now trying it before approaching a personal physician for a recommendation. Participating physicians (5 of 12), coalesce that, "It's nice to have that [adult use] system, at least for getting people started." Each express, how "surprised," they've been, "at how many patients have tried it through a recreational dispensary before going to his or her regular doctor." Unfortunately, they also share, "Of course, they come to me after that doctor denies them. But, at least, now the doctor denying them is referring them to a physician who can help." "It's progress," as another acknowledges, "but, it's slow progress."

Within stories, physicians in these states (5 of 12) also note that,

"This new [*recreational*] system helped attract patients to medical cannabis therapy that had never used cannabis before. In these states, a patient over the age of 21, has the chance to try it legally, before deciding about using it medicinally and starting the cumbersome process of registering."

A physician in Washington avows,

> *Because we have a legal cannabis system as well, for adult use and I'm pretty much only seeing adults, I can and often do recommend. I tell patients that this is something that they should consider trying. I give them some guidance on what might be a good way to start...They don't need any paperwork from me to go and access it at an adult use store in the city.*

The ability "to send a patient to try it *before* they have to jump through 200 hoops is a godsend."

Participating physicians in these states, and those practicing in Integrative Cannabis practices in other states (8 of 12), each conveyed that they were receiving more "undercover" referrals from local physicians. This is good business for Integrative Cannabis physicians, but costly for chronically and terminally ill patients. Regardless, three-quarters of the physician participants (8 of 12) stated they thought, "Legalization can help to take the stigma away." An Oregon physician acknowledges,

> *Now that all adults over 21 can use cannabis without being labeled a criminal they have begun asking their doctors about it. Their regular doctors often refer them to me and send their records right over. But, they never note in the patient's chart they've done this. I find that interesting. I've gone from black sheep to trusted referral source though I am the same doctor I've always been.*

These changes in laws regarding adult use of cannabis have increased medicinal consumption.

Relayed as a Colorado physician shares her story,

> *We started seeing more and more people coming to the clinic who had never used it before after the law legalizing cannabis in Colorado was passed. Because before it was illegal for adults if you didn't have a medical card. By definition, if you tried marijuana, you were a criminal. People aren't, even if they tried it, they wouldn't...for so many people the stigma is very large. It's very large. It's very hard for them to come in. For some people...it's very limiting. Because they don't want me to put something in their chart. Then they get a knock at the door or something... it really worries some people. They don't want to be a criminal. They don't want to be on the wrong side of the law. Being able to even raise the question is so much easier for people because they know it's legal for them to use it as an adult. Since then we've just seen more people come and be willing to try it. In the great majority of cases they get the result, they get help, and they come back. They are able to use it and their lives are improving.*

Although some of the physicians view decriminalization or "legalization" positively, others, though they recommend its use, still have prohibitionist concerns about the "recreational" initiatives. A physician in private practice explains the ingrained belief in society and within the medical community (LL) from his own perspective,

> *Everybody realizes that to a certain degree people look at medical marijuana as just a way to get the door open for legalization for recreational use. I think that's part of the anxiety about physicians getting involved with the cannabis treatments.*

Another shares,

> *The state headed in the wrong direction with recreational marijuana because they are only interested in the tax revenues it will bring in. It is generating a lot of revenue. The program is only going to keep expanding. But I think it's going to be to the detriment of the medical program.*

An Oregon physician shares,

> *A lot of the patients are speculating that the state really wants to drive out the medical program and just put everybody under recreational. They can make more tax money that way. We'll see, time will tell. I've talked to some physicians up in Washington and they say the medical dispensaries are closing there.*

Physicians (5 of 12) credit patient advocates for sustaining medical cannabis programs "despite political threats and pervasive myths about stoners." Again, physicians recommending cannabis realize that because medical cannabis is effective, "It's not a joke. It's not a cover to get legalization, because that's the assumption. It's just a way to get people a substance legally that they're already using recreationally, but not really medically."

As patient participants in adult use states (7 of 20) conveyed as they shared stories,

"There are a lot of patients that are accessing our recreational system for medicinal reasons. There are a wide-variety of reasons why they're not on that medical list, but they are using medicinally."

As well, two additional patients share, "Before I decided whether I would ask my doctor for a recommendation or register as a patient, I went to Colorado and tried it." For each, "That one week vacation convinced me it was worth a try." A Colorado patient, who also advocates for patient rights, shares how she's responded to numerous "allegations or accusations that the reason Colorado's medical program is growing since legalization is so people can avoid the higher sales tax (27-36% vs 8.25% on average, for example per Colorado.gov).

"Wait a minute, these aren't just people that want to get high and avoid sales tax. I've heard that argument a hundred times! No! These are patients."

In accordance with state regulations in Colorado, one must be a registered cannabis patient meeting minimum qualifications. For example, they must be suffering from a qualifying condition for which a physician recommends medical cannabis as an option.

Participating physicians (5 of 12) in states that have enacted 'adult use' or decriminalization initiatives also discuss attempts to "remove medical marijuana programs once legalization occurs." An Integrative Cannabis physician in Colorado shares the following as part of her story of becoming an advocate for patients because of the "quality-of-life" improvements she's witnessed since she began working in this arena.

> *There were forces in the state or voices in the state, including those high up in the medical administration, that would rather there not be a medical marijuana program. They were like 'This is ridiculous. We need to close this program.' Insinuating it was out of control or something. The way they would do it would be through the doctors because you can destroy the medical marijuana industry if no more doctors will write recommendations. If there are no recommendations, there are*

no patients, the dispensaries go out of business. It is really that simple! There was pressure being applied at that very moment to doctors, because they're the gatekeepers under the law. They wanted the recreational to take off. They were like, 'Make everybody pay the taxes...there's recreational now, what do you need medical for?'

Patients have also felt the "push-back from state medical programs following decriminalization" of adult cannabis use. A Washington patient said, "As soon as legalization was passed, the state went after the medical program." In similar ways, embedded in the following story, a Colorado patient shares,

Since we decriminalized adult use, this state has tried to chip away at the medical program. They think they'll get more tax money by pushing everyone to adult use, but instead the black market gets more customers.

For both parties, these "two separate policy issues are terribly intertwined and have wreaked havoc on the weak medical cannabis systems we now rely on," a Colorado physician conveys.

Medical Cannabis Refugees

Because *cannabis sativa* remains a Schedule I Controlled Substance nationwide and only 28 of our 50 states have medical cannabis programs in effect, the phenomena of medical cannabis refugee has become an unexpected consequence of medicalization.

A *medical cannabis refugee* is a chronically or terminally ill patient who has relocated to a medical cannabis or a decriminalized state, *specifically* to use cannabis as medication.

The predominance of this phenomenon has increased dramatically in the last few years, as witness by participants. Of the patients participating in this study more than half (13 of 20) are medical cannabis refugees; after relocating to register as a medical cannabis patient in a state they moved to specifically because it provided them access to a medical cannabis program. As a New Mexico patient voices,

> We moved here because I deal with a tremendous amount of pain. I was on a lot of narcotics. In fact, a 27-year old friend of ours passed away after taking the medications I was on. My son was already living here and he just freaked out. 'Mom, you have got to get here!'

Another medical cannabis refugee shares,

> My doctor in Mississippi said, "There is nothing more we can do for you, you might want to consider going to Colorado and seeing if anyone there can help." I researched it and we moved. Now a year later, I am cancer-free...and staying in Colorado!

A U.S. military veteran showing "severe symptoms from Gulf War Syndrome" shares his experience, which was more embattled than anticipated,

> Here I had made a move halfway across the country just to be told that I wasn't allowed to use it [by a Veteran's Administration physician]. It made me feel like I was a criminal. They actually told me that they could stop any treatments or medication I was on if they wanted to if I kept using cannabis.

As another cannabis refugee and advocate shares her story she voices,

> We've known a lot of families that have relocated here for cannabis therapy. Unfortunately, a lot of them uproot with the wrong information or thinking it will be easy to qualify. It's not

easy, it's a hard program to get in. The biggest hurdle is
finding a doctor to recommend. If you have a sick child, which
most of these refugees do, well then, it takes two doctors.
That's a lot of time and expense for a family with a disabled
child. If they can find two doctors to recommend.

This growing problem is directly linked to the Schedule I status of cannabis federally and will be discussed further in Chapter Five.

LL: Interior Collective

An integral evaluation of a metanarrative, where basic commonalities and relationships become more apparent among a multiplicity of perspectives and the expectations of doctor-patient relationships (UR), provides insight into the culture of control (LL) as described by study participants.

"We've been told that this is socially unacceptable."

The following section contains metanarrative of participants based on LL themes within shared stories.

Culture of Control

As described in Chapter Two, common language, signs, and symbols that are understood and shared among humans characterize the LL quadrant. To successfully rescript cultural beliefs about what it means to be a cannabis patient or to recommend cannabis as a medical therapy, a reflection on participant experience in this area is insightful. The taboos, rituals, and shared meanings about cannabis that participants discuss most prevalently regard cultural and professional stigma or loss of status (Goffman, 1963, Cummings and Cummings, 1965) linked directly to ingrained social constructs and a lack of education on the subject matter. However, before drilling down into these critical issues, an examination of language is necessitated.

Language is Culture

Stigmatizing language, like that used to develop social constructs (LL), is internalized and can be marginalizing (UL). Both patient and physician narratives contain traces of LL social myths and stereotypes. "I grew up in a very conservative community. It was known as the devil weed there." Every narrative (32 of 32) contained stigmatizing references that had been internalized by or projected upon others by both parties: Stoner, pot-head, weed, pot and laziness were the most referenced (296 references in 32 interviews). A Colorado patient says of his doctors, "They just have a picture of a patient with a joint burning." Overall, participants believe (32 of 32) that "goes back to a lack of education" (LL/LR) and it is a constant battle for both parties that will be discussed in further detail in Chapter Five.

Though both parties are amid a language change, moving outside the cannabis community and away from those educated about the matter, most define cannabis via slang (marijuana or other terms) in order that they be understood. This type of language is stigmatizing in any community and can be internalized (UL) as will be described later in the study. Three of the participating physicians (3 of 12) had particularly stigmatizing language shadowing his or her own narrative. Interestingly all three of the physicians are practicing within hospital or clinic systems. As well, they are the physicians that did not demonstrate a transformative learning experience as described later in this chapter. Sample references include:

- Even the potheads who smoke marijuana to get high...
- Then there is the whole *reefer madness* from the 30's and 40's...but a lot of people do just like getting high.
- I still think that marijuana users are some of the stupidest people I've ever met.

These examples demonstrate that there is still much work to be done in this arena.

Patients (16 of 20) described "language immersion" journeys into the "medical science of cannabis." An Illinois patient conveys,

> *The language, the terminology - these are things that have a
> learning curve. For me - as a patient - to be explaining a bodily
> system, receptors, and cannabinoids, that's a lot of information
> to take in.*

Another Illinois patient voices,

> *You'd think my doctors would appreciate the effort I've put into
> learning about this and try to learn some of the language too.
> My primary asked me, 'How's the pot working for you?' That's
> not very respectful.*

Patient participants (12 of 20) have the expectation that physicians will understand the terminology used, whether it is scientific (i.e. endocannabinoid system, cannabinoids, cannabidiol, etc.) or communal (i.e. weed, pot, joint, bong rip, dab, edible, etc.) and believe "these terms should be the part of education programs offered to medical professionals, not just doctors, and the public." As a Connecticut patient illustrates,

> *Doctors need to know what bong rips are and that they can
> provide a huge relief for pain issues. For me, bong rips are a
> healthy option in comparison to the OxyContin and Fentanyl
> that they helped me reduce, then stop taking completely within
> 6 months of cannabis therapy. I mean, I use cannabis oil as my
> main medicine, but a bong rip will just step me away from the
> pain so that I can handle it.*

More about how language can be stigmatizing will be discussed in Chapter Five.

Drug Use & Abuse: Myths that Stigmatize

Perhaps social stigma regarding the use of illicit, Schedule I drugs is "one of the greatest obstacles" for either patients or physicians "to get over." The collective judgement that "people like to get high" has taken on a negative, condemnatory tone, over the past three generations and is a large piece of the dominant narrative reinforcing the message that "cannabis is bad." One of the private practice physicians espouses the dominant narrative,

> *It's just another way to escape. Some people use alcohol, some people use marijuana, some people use narcotics. It's just a mind-altering substance and people really like those.*

Several other physicians (5 of 12) and several patients (6 of 20) have the shadow narrative of "people like the escape from life and sometimes are abusing it because of that" embedded within his or her own testimony.

Myths about getting high are so prolific that they influence treatment. Two of the physician participants (2 of 12) noted that they prescribe Suboxone to medical cannabis patients they've recommended for "to help them handle the euphoria" and "avoid addiction." Chapter Five will elaborate on this counter-indicated treatment. As the patient-naturopath describes,

> *One of the things that some of the doctors are concerned about, and this is based on misinformation and stigma, is that the patient is going to become an addict; a marijuana addict. That's all they've ever heard; it is addictive. Doctors still, believe me, they are not by any means or in any place right now where they're very supportive.*

Another patient voices that she conceals (UR) her cannabis use from her physician because of she fears this type of internalized stigmatization (UL) for them both,

> *I didn't tell that doctor what I was doing on my own. It is because they can feel uncomfortable, not that I want to hide it. I wish I could openly discuss it with them but they make me feel like I'm some sort of criminal or drug addict. I don't want to*

put myself through that! I don't want to put them through it
either!

She goes on to share, "There is a lot of prejudice within the medical community about cannabis. They generally think people are just abusing it."

The issue of cannabis use is one of diversity and participating patients (12 of 12) believe with education, many doctors can "come to accept this as not a drug of abuse, but a better, safer option for many." But they also share, "We're not there yet." Why? In several patient's opinion,

> *It is the bedside manner of the doctors. They need to learn how*
> *to talk to their patients about cannabis. It's the same thing*
> *about parents being able to learn how to talk about it without*
> *making it feel weird. We've grown up making the conversation*
> *about drugs weird and uncomfortable. Now cannabis is being*
> *used as a day-to-day regimen for a lot of sick people.*

Education -"or the lack thereof - is the cornerstone to making change. You don't know what change to make if you haven't learned anything about it."

Loss of Status

Each of the physician participants (12 of 12) recognized that they would be learning from his or her patients when they first provided a medical cannabis recommendation. "I didn't know anything about it when patients first asked me for a recommendation." In many different ways, they expressed they are "humbled by the opportunity to learn about this from so many vantage points." However, loss of status and discriminatory experiences have been a part of the recommendation process, particularly within the local medical community (LL), among peers (LL/UR), and within medical corporations (LR). "I am now seen as being outside the organization's company culture." Each of these cultures, including peer relationships (LL/UR) are influenced by LR policies and practices, as well as LL myths, taboos, and societal stigma, but cause UL effect.

An Oregon physician shares the following experiences,

> When I started to practice in 2014, it wasn't long after that I received a letter from the director of [County Medical Professional Organization]. It is an organization of doctors in my county. This letter basically told me to cease and desist treating their patients because "we want no part of this." I've been the black sheep in the medical community here since then.

A Washington doctor voices,

> It's really part of the structural violence or structural indifference to cannabis from the federal health sector, because I worked for a government hospital...there was all the more taboo and restriction.

He goes on to share,

> The ethics person at the hospital wasn't even willing to sit down over a cup of coffee and talk about this. I worked against that and tried to find ways to talk to the people who ran the place.

The main reason patients use medical cannabis evaluation centers is to avoid losing status with his or her personal physicians.

"I didn't feel confident that my own physician would be willing to give me a recommendation. I was also very hesitant to have that on my medical records, which actually proved to be a wise approach."

Since registering as a patient, a considerable number of the patient participants, (7 of

20) have not engaged in a conversation or shared the medical cannabis status with a personal primary care or specialty doctor with the support of an evaluation center or Integrative Cannabis physician. For several (4 of 7), they were "ignored" or "refused" a recommendation from a primary or specialty physician, so they "see no need to bring the subject back up." A Colorado patient shares,

> *I did what I had to do, I went to a marijuana doctor and got my recommendation. I asked [my primary care doctor] about it once and she wouldn't talk with me. Why should I tell her now? She should ask. But, she won't because she doesn't want to hear that it's helping me.*

The expertise and embodied knowledge that this patient should share has found deaf ears (UR) and her fears cause internalized suffering (UL).

Marginalization occurs when patients are punished for requesting treatment challenging the norm (LL) or the expert (UR). Unfortunately, this is the case for many patients. The following narratives were shared by patients in Colorado and Washington, two states not only with medical cannabis policies, but decriminalized adult use policies. A Washington patient experiences,

> *Being fired from a doctor's practice is humiliating, it has happened to me twice and I've quit two other practices because of the doctor's obvious ignorance about this subject.*

A Colorado patient shares,

> *A few months after I received my recommendation, I went to one of my regular doctors and told her how much better I was doing since this change. For the next 30-minutes, the most time she's ever taken with me, I received a lecture on the dangers of cannabis. Due to that fact, I don't talk to my doctors about medical cannabis anymore. They have no idea why my health is improving.*

Patients are unrecognized experts within the medical cannabis arena, because of their embodied knowledge and experience (UL). Instead of fearing or experiencing a loss of status for inquiring about medical cannabis therapies, physician participants (8 of 12) specializing in Integrative Cannabis practices recognize "patients are a wealth of valuable information about this subject." Yet, for patients it is difficult to decide whether to even risk asking a personal physician for a recommendation. A Minnesota patient shares,

> I was apprehensive of approaching my doctor because I was scared about his reaction to it. I knew it was helping but I didn't know if he would listen.

Who's the Expert in the Doctor-Patient Relationship?

After a patient "survives the state's registry challenges" (LR) and gets access to medical cannabis (LR), they may become empowered "to take responsibility for my own healthcare" (UL/UR). This response often challenges the LL myth that the physician is the expert in medical therapies, as the *controller*, while patients are the *receivers* of the doctor's expertise and the prescribed treatment. An Illinois patient conveys,

> In the conversations, I've had with my physicians, it has been me explaining it to them, instead of them explaining it to me.

Another Illinois patient shares,

> Part of the rolling of their eyes and rejecting it right off the bat is because they don't know about it. They forget that the patients are the ones living in their bodies actually dealing with it. We research it and then feel comfortable enough to experiment with it. If they researched it, like I have, they'd be much more comfortable with it.

Culturally and collectively, as one physician notes, it is "a little hard for us doctors to swallow the fact that the patient is one up on us here." For that reason, it isn't hard to understand that patients find,

"In my experience, doctors don't really like their patients knowing more than they do."

This certainly represents a disorienting dilemma for both parties. Yet, patients have UR expectations within LL healthcare communities. What patient participants seem to asking for is an opportunity for co-decision-making in healthcare decisions. This study will explore co-decision-making further in Chapter Five.

Patients educating physicians is a cultural shift within traditional U.S. medical communities, as well as for patients who have been taught to view doctors collectively as experts. However, for the patient participants who have overcome so many obstacles to become a cannabis patient and experienced a positive therapeutic outcome, educating a personal physician, engaging in co-decision-making, and working alongside the doctor is empowering. A Colorado patient shares her empowering story,

> *My primary care doctor was actually curious to see how it works for me. I was giving her feedback on what I was doing and on what I was trying. Essentially, I was my own Guinea pig. That's how I started with edibles. Edibles have a longer-lasting effect for me, so the spasticity was gone longer. Then, I started eating edibles from the dispensaries; that's how I started gauging the milligrams, the THC and the CBD Once the CBD craze came I tried using CBD only for my spasticity. It doesn't work! I have to have THC I've found the levels I need for my body. It's taken a while but now I can find relief!*

A Colorado patient explains how she "surprises" her doctors,

> *I love explaining to my doctors that I use cannabis mainly by*

topical salve. 'Topical? Really? Does that get you high?' No, it doesn't get me high, but it does get me out of my wheelchair!

However, as an Arizona patient observes,

It is really hard when you're the one educating them; yet, you have questions that you need answers to. Doctors want to help but they don't have the education or information they need. They're uncomfortable because of this, so it is easier to just say, "No."

Holistic vs. Western Collective Ideologies

In the LL quadrant, it is important to consider the cultural differences between holistic healthcare and conventional western (U.S.) healthcare, as it was discussed by nearly every participant (29 of 32). The participating physicians (8 of 12) repeatedly remarked that "my approach" is holistic "in comparison" with LR medical institutions and "normal healthcare communities." The other participating physicians (4 of 12) affirm a "holistic mindset differs" from the norm. Traditional healthcare communities are heavily laden in allopathic culture. A contrast between these approaches is shared in Chapter Five.

Participating patients (16 of 20) specifically state they prefer a holistic approach and "don't understand" the collective resistance to it from the U.S. medical community (LL), institutions (LR), or insurance companies (LR). An Arizona patient voices,

There is a reluctance to treat the patient with a holistic approach; where they take the entire person, body, mind and all the systems that make it up and put equal emphasis on it and take it into consideration when making a diagnosis, proposing a treatment, or even evaluating how the treatments are working.

A Colorado patient conveys,

> *Western medicine has become so formulaic 'If you have this*
> *problem, prescribe this pill, if you have a side-effect have a*
> *second pill.' In order to help patients, we need to move away*
> *from that formulaic approach, which does take more time:*
> *where the doctor spends more time with the patient, talking to*
> *the patient, understanding what's going on, and thinking about*
> *what kind of factors could be contributing to a particular*
> *situation.*

This study will discuss these and other factors more in depth in the section on Transformative Learning and in Chapter Five.

Cultural Shifts: Pharmacy to Dispensary

The primary support proffered by the physician for cannabis therapy is the recommendation; rarely is it supplied along with education, consultation, or referral to a social service agency. Participating physicians (10 of 12) note that the dispensary model is also outside the norm for the medical community and "is hard for the medical community to accept." For several (3 of 10) this cultural shift "is hard to swallow." An Illinois physician shares,

> *To me it seems one step above drug dealer, the patient doesn't*
> *have medical professionals to help them.*

Another voices,

> *It's frustrating to send patients to a dispensary with very little*
> *information to go on. They often end up buying products they*
> *don't need or want. These dispensary employees aren't*
> *counselors. They are salespeople.*

The testimony of participating patients (18 of 20) supports the physician's comments about the collective failings of dispensaries. Several report, "I knew more than the associate [at the dispensary], which was crazy." A New Mexico patient shares her frustration with dispensary models,

> On my first trip to a dispensary, I knew what I wanted:
> cannabis oil. I had to explain to the first dispensary what it
> was - this was in 2012. I ended up explaining it to all 15
> dispensaries in the state. It's now 2016, I find it highly doubtful
> that even one of these dispensaries has it in stock. I learned
> how to make my own.

Another patient, who is employed within the cannabis industry voices,

> Dispensaries are not being responsible to the community. They
> aren't honest about the way they grow or produce products
> and they don't educate themselves or others on cannabis.
> They're one step from the black market, they are not really
> medical because society has culturally ostracized them. They
> don't think they have an obligation to the community that
> stigmatizes them. It's a terrible cycle of ignorance and
> irresponsibility.

Other patients (3 of 20) through personal search found "respite" and "education" at local dispensaries; each admitting "it was quite a search to find one I was comfortable at." An Arizona patient shares about his "favorite dispensary,"

> You are able to use and borrow books and DVDs. You can
> socialize with other cannabis patients. They made a space
> where you relax and create relationships. The other places are
> just like normal dispensaries, you walk in, there is a waiting
> room, and you walk in, pick your medicine and go. [Name of
> dispensary] is just a place you get a warmer feeling. You feel
> like you are in community. They are accepting of everyone. It is
> really a wonderful place to learn and be with others.

Unfortunately, this type of experience is rare, per shared patient stories.

Lack of Social Support

Physician participants (5 of 12) commented that "When I realized that the patient had been in discussion with someone about using medical marijuana, it helped." These comments came because the researcher runs an educational non-profit organization that educates patients and physicians on the use of cannabis, as disclosed earlier. The eCS Therapy Center is among the first to operate as a social service agency for medical cannabis patients. The patient-naturopath provides similar services to patients within her state via an evaluation center model. As a New Mexico patient describes the naturopath's practice, he says, "It is 200% better than any other service in the state." However, as most patient participants (12 of 20) recognize, "Besides your organization, I don't know anyone else working with patients that doesn't own a dispensary" or "isn't being paid by one to pimp their products." With no state funding and no support coming from within the cannabis industry, the model of social service agency that doctors and patients both recognize is sorely in need, but difficult to sustain.

Cannabis education organizations perform services within a community that physicians and patients find helpful, as the patient-naturopath does. It is the hope of both parties (32 of 32) that "services like these that educate and reach out within the community become the next focus of policymakers" (LR). As one doctor states,

"The medical community and culture is used to having social service support for patients suffering all kinds of conditions, given the unique nature of bringing a medicine back from illegal to legal should certainly justify social support for patients and their physicians."

Patients shared the importance of social support being combined with medical care. A Colorado patient shares,

Our doctor referred us to [name of public advocate]. That was the most generous thing she could have done. She couldn't write a recommendation but her referral to [name of advocate] was priceless.

As mentioned earlier in this section, as a patient it can often be difficult to find support and the information you need to use cannabis therapies successfully. The "undercover referrals" to a recommending physician by a primary care physician helped four patient participants (4 of 20) find the support they'd been searching for.

Patient expertise is self-learned through a combination of internet searches, conversations with other patients, and embodied knowledge. All twenty (20 of 20) patient participants discussed in-depth online research that they had conducted prior to seeking a recommendation for medical cannabis, including the PubMed information shared earlier. Three (3 of 20) patient participants noted that they graduated from a renown cannabis education program in California: Oaksterdam. All three are employed within the cannabis industry. Twelve (12) other patients noted some type of workshop, educational event, or self-led cannabis event involving education or awareness as vital to his or her learning process. "I learned just as much spending time in community between workshops as I did in the classes." All patient participants (20 of 20) shared personal research efforts in the same manner physicians did. For example, one patient states, "I believe I might be eligible for a Google degree in cannabinoids given how many hours I've spent online reading scientific studies." And a physician shared,

"I believe Google should begin offering a cannabinoid specialty, not only would I qualify but most of my patients have spent as many, if not more, hours online reading clinical data as I have."

Family and Community Acceptance

The issue of how we view drug use in this country (LL) combined with the (LR) Controlled Substance status of cannabis sativa assures that cannabis use affects family and community acceptance. Current UR issues with militarized law enforcement and the enormous social impact of abandoning mental health support and substance abuse funding collide (LR) to affect stigmatic social impact in the LL quadrant. A Washington physician shares on this issue,

> *It really is so variable. The responses vary by demographics. It really is a demographic thing because it is different age groups, immigrant groups, and ethnic origins. They've experienced different messaging about cannabis from a young age until now. You have to be ready for anything.*

A Nevada doctor voices,

> *So many patients come to me and they say they have to use cannabis secretly because other family members don't approve or think they're going to get into trouble. The misinformation out there is mind-boggling and it is so ingrained in people! The 70 plus years of nonsense causes a lot of patients to use it secretly, even hiding it from their own family.*

Several of the patient participants (5 of 20) noted that in addition to having a doctor-patient relationship with the patient, the doctor is also "in charge of" the healthcare of other family members. Some (3 of 5) mentioned this as reason for withholding his or her cannabis patient status with a primary physician. For each, it was a point worthy of discussion. For one, it presents an ideal scenario between a "previously undecided" physician and a patient "focused on medical cannabis" alternatives,

> *The doctor that I have now, has been my family doctor, my dad's, my mother's, my grandmother's doctor for the last ten*

years. The last 12 years for my parents; the last four years for me. I've always felt really comfortable telling her everything. I never had a problem or even second thoughts about talking to her about cannabis. What I'd been talking to her about was getting off of the Flexural. That was one thing that was really important to me, and that happened! She has always been very supportive. I guess, not overly supportive, but she does ask how I use it. We did have the conversation about smoking. I told her that I now vape more than I smoke and it used to be vice versa. She seems to be up-to-date with the information I am giving her...I had an injury last December. It was almost like a paralysis in the right arm, having to do with some nerve damage in the neck. I had gone into an Urgent Care. They had prescribed me hydrocodone and naproxen. I thought, 'This is exactly what I needed; they diagnosed the situation.' I had been on those for about a week when I went to my primary care physician. She said, 'I need you to get off those because you said you were primarily using cannabis as your pain thing.' I said, 'You know, you're right.' I went and found the strongest cannabis tincture. I was buying those and taking those, every night for my pain. I was able to get up in the morning. Unlike the first week when I stayed in bed all day. The hydrocodone and naproxen just made me - I just wanted to say in bed. I had no energy whatsoever...Working with my doctor and letting her know how I was using it within my regimen really was a big help... With this injury, I also needed to work with a nerve doctor and a physical therapist. Both were on-board with my decision. The neurologist told me that 'Along with the physical therapy and steroid injections we'll have you better and back to normal.' I said, 'Maybe the physical therapy part, but I am not taking steroids.' The physical therapy went a little bit longer than expected. It was supposed to be six months, it ended up

being eight months, but that was fine with me. Working with
the doctors and letting them know that this is my choice - that
this is what I'm taking for the pain - I am doing it this way! It
was very empowering.

Equally divided in experiences, patient participants (10 of 20) share stigmatizing situations with family members and the other half (10 of 20) find "more support within my family than I'd ever expected." Interestingly, the outcome had no gender bias, in that half of each group was male, half female, meaning there was no discernable difference in expectations about how family would treat the patient based on gender, in this study's findings. A Connecticut patient attests,

When I first started using cannabis only a few of my family
members knew. It wasn't a big deal but they did stereotype it.

A New Mexico patient shares,

My own family is so bent on believing what the medical doctors
say that they won't use medical cannabis because some doctor
convinced them that it is bad for them.

On the other hand, an Illinois patient reports,

They've all been supportive of me. I've talked to my pastor. I've
talked to other people...I don't care who you are, I will walk
right up and tell you. 'Look at me! I don't eat a bunch of fucking
pills anymore! My kidneys aren't dying! That's great news,
isn't it?'

Time after time,

"Patients worry about talking to their family or a religious organization, *until they find out how it helps.*

Once they've experienced it, they become much more open about discussing it with these entities."

Embodied knowledge empowers.

Because cannabis sativa has been illicit for nearly 80 years and remains a CSA Schedule I substance, generational issues within families often affect understanding and acceptance. "The reefer madness mentality is very strong still, especially with older people." As an Illinois patient relays, "It's been illicit my grandmother's entire life, how is she supposed to know the truth?" Improved educational support regarding cannabis use would help change occur, as will be discussed in Chapter Five.

UR: Exterior Individual

Despite growing evidence that the endocannabinoid system (eCS) is vital to human health, *cannabis sativa* remains classified under the U.S. Controlled Substances Act as a Schedule I Substance (LR). Both physicians and patients interested in exploring this therapy through state-approved medical cannabis programs frequently encounter resistance or confusion from the other party; particularly when it comes to the actual recommendation of cannabis. This portion of the study explores the social ramifications of the Controlled Substances Act's Schedule I status of *cannabis sativa* as the data reflect within the UR quadrant. LR and LL issues such as political power-as-dominance, knowledge control, social violence, and cultural beliefs directly affect the doctor-patient relationship and communication experience (UR). Sometimes patients conceal cannabis use in response. A Connecticut patient conveys,

> *I've been a cannabis patient for four years and I've never once mentioned it to any of my regular doctors. I just don't want to deal with them. They really have no idea why I am getting better.*

A Colorado patient shares why he conceals his cannabis patient status from his doctor,

> *It's simple: I just don't want to have this conversation with my doctor. I don't know how he will respond.*

Of the twelve physicians (12) participating in this study, eight (8 of 12) operate or are employed within an Integrative Cannabis practice, as noted earlier. The other four (4 of 12) physicians work within large medical systems. Regardless, all (12 of 12) admit "getting past fears, institutional concerns, and gaining a comfort level with cannabis has been a journey." However, only two of the physicians practicing in medical institutes (2 of 12) recommend cannabis "regularly" without prompting by patients. The other two physicians (2 of 12) "have so far felt more comfortable with patients initiating the conversation."

Participating physicians (12 of 12) share that the uneasy part was saying "I really have no experience in being able to tell you how effective this might be, how helpful it will be. This is a relatively new modality of treatment for your condition." They also agree,

"Part of it is being on the treatment journey with the patient and physician both learning as we go along."

The openness to "cannabis use as an issue of diversity that we can learn more about and find acceptance for is vital to patients interacting with regular medical professionals." Participating physicians (8 of 12) also share similar experiences and perceptions,

> *Medical cannabis isn't going away. It is here to stay because it works so well for so many things. It was because my patients shared their stories that I came to understand and was forced to more research. Seeing it help people - being open to seeing it help people - that changes ideologies. As a group and as individuals, physicians need to be open to observing patients*

who choose this option. They may come to find themselves recommending it to other patients. That's what happened with me.

Another physician observes,

> *As patients are willing to be brave and talk to the doctors about it...and now, more people are willing because of how much change they've experienced.*

Another shares how her "thinking changed,"

> *If patients can have that dialogue with doctors, even those who aren't or don't feel willing to do the recommendation - and there are a number of reasons for that - it's not just that they might not be willing to do it, it may be that they can't do it, but are very curious about it, it can change things between the doctor and the patient in a positive way. That's what helped me change my thinking about this.*

Unfortunately, finding this type of support outside of a medical cannabis evaluation center or even within one is rare. Instead, as patient participants affirm (14 of 20), they frequently face traumatizing and stigmatic experiences when they approach personal physicians regarding a medical cannabis recommendation. A California patient conveys, "I had to fire my primary over using cannabis. He just wouldn't listen to me." And, as a Connecticut patient shares,

> *There are times when you need to talk to your regular doctor...once you let that out of the bag, it's something that sticks with you as a patient. Once the doctors realize that you use cannabis as medicine first, you get a different treatment, that's for sure.*

In total, nine participating patients (9 of 20) mention "firing" a physician. In only two participating patient cases (2 of 20), did the primary or specialty physician provide the patient's medical cannabis recommendation as a part of a regular office visit. In only these two cases (10% of patient participants), did a study participant obtain a recommendation *within* his or her normal healthcare system. One Illinois patient had an experience that differed greatly from others,

> *It wasn't something I went to ask for, it was something I saw at the office that they were already offering. I happened to ask and he said I was qualified. Of course, I was excited because I knew then that I would not have to keep dodging the alleys to get the medicine that worked for me.*

Often, participating patients (16 of 20) obtained a recommendation but received little support or education, only receiving true evaluation services, "a review of my records, a few questions and a signature on a form, all for $200."

Another sign that individual physicians are bucking medical systems (LR) and cultures (LL), both physician and patient participants note that Integrative Cannabis physicians are receiving more "undercover referrals" from local physicians than in the past, as mentioned earlier. Particularly, participants in Washington and Colorado (10 of 32) all noted this change, sharing that changes in laws regarding adult use (decriminalization initiatives) have "opened awareness for both physicians and patients," as communicated in the LL quadrant discussion. A Colorado physician shares,

> *I hear from some of our recommending physicians that they are getting referrals from a lot of these other doctors. Those that can't recommend because they're restricted by their hospital or their health care network. For whatever reason, they just don't feel like they are knowledgeable enough to make that call, but they are sending people to medical cannabis doctors.*

The reasons that patients do not engage a personal doctor in a conversation about a medical cannabis recommendation or its use are myriad and often difficult to untangle. However, the physician's "bedside manner" or "willingness to listen before judging" are prime factors that are being considered by patients. Unfortunately, patients may be too "intimidated" or "afraid" to engage with his or her doctor simply due to behavioral concerns. As an Arizona patient exclaims,

> *The doctor just spewed inaccurate information. I found myself*
> *correcting her and she was pulling the 'I'm a doctor' card.*
> *[Patient scoffs] We parted ways.*

She goes on to share,

> *Some patients are intimidated by their doctor because of the*
> *doctor's authoritarian personality. I won't deal with that*
> *anymore.*

Behaviors or even perceived behaviors affect UR interactions. A physician shares how a doctor's stigmatizing behavior may affect patients without cannabis experience,

> *A lot of patients have great intention and have a lot of great*
> *information; they're probably on the right track. Then they go*
> *to their regular doctor and let a little bit slip out. The doctor*
> *might destroy all their hopes and bring them down to the point*
> *where they might not even want to go forward with cannabis*
> *treatment.*

Study participants, both physicians and patients (32 of 32) commented on the importance of teaching communication skills that "open the doctor-patient relationship to improved discussions" about disorienting dilemmas like this, as will be discussed in Chapter Five.

UL: Interior Individual

The Upper-Left (UL) quadrant references the interior reality lived by a person. Schwartz (2013) describes the UL quadrant as "posited as the locus of the master or key hermeneutic arena of perspectives; or, in greater balance, the lens through which the other quadrants are seen, interpreted, and evaluated" (p. 169). This quadrant encompasses a person's subjective personal experience, as the following narratives share. Internalized guilt, fear, or stigma has significant effect on well-being and personal decision-making in this quadrant, as demonstrated within participant stories.

Internalized Language

The euphoria-factor of cannabis use or "the high" is the most stigmatized aspect of the plant. However, after some experience with patients using cannabis or cannabis use themselves, most participants (30 of 32; 20 patients, 10 physicians) acknowledged the medicinal and UL value to the euphoric experience. A patient examines his experience,

> "I may experience a little *euphoria* occasionally, is that horrible? It gave me a sense of well-being."

Several physicians (6 of 12) and patients (15 of 20) share, "That step back from pain or discomfort is important to the patient." Others share disbelief and frustration with the effects of these myths. A Colorado patient voices,

> *Given how many anti-depressants and anti-anxiety drugs we*
> *are legally prescribed and how much alcohol is consumed in*
> *our country, it is surprising to have so many people concerned*
> *about the high of cannabis.*

For some, the reality of the experience is far different from the myths to which they've been exposed. One patient described her first experience using cannabis,

> *I'd never been high before, never used marijuana. I was scared*
> *to death. When I tried the tincture for the first time and felt*

that high, *well, it was the first time I relaxed or felt halfway human in years. It was not what I expected or had been told I should fear.*

Isolation

Chronically and terminally ill people often become isolated. "As a patient, when you don't feel well you can't get things done. You stay home. Days turn into weeks, weeks into months, months into years." Nearly all the patient participants (18 of 20) shared that isolation "had a particularly negative effect on their quality-of-life," at some point during a health struggle. In fact, seven patients (7 of 20) specifically shared that this isolation "helped me conceal my cannabis use. When I started coming back to life, my friends and family were shocked to learn cannabis had unlocked my door to fellowship, so to speak." As another patient shares, "When you are alone, it is hard to have hope." But he goes on to say,

"When you feel better you start *doing*. You get re-engaged with life."

Participating patients (19 of 20) affirm that, collectively, they share similar experiences. As voiced by one patient,

> *As I started to feel better I became more active. I also spent more time thinking about my cannabis use, both current and past. I came to see I needed to get much more focused on how I was using it so that I would continue to experience improvement. That's what I did, I got really focused and my health greatly improved. I got my life back.*

Patients with previous cannabis experience also share that "I didn't realize I was a medical user." As an Arizona patient conveys,

I was a recreational user for decades before I got sick and
became a cannabis patient. It was after I became a patient that
I started to realize all my use had been medicinal in nature:
stress, anxiety, aches and pains, migraines, I had always been
using it medically.

All the patient participants (20 of 20) depicted personal current cannabis use with a descriptive statement at some point in the interview. Not one described the casual use of cannabis. Each, in fact, described *focused* use.

"My use quit being casual and started being serious."

In fact, most (11 of 20) think of medical use as excluding casual or recreational use. As one patient shares,

There are two different types of factions of marijuana users in
this country. There are medical marijuana patients and there
are recreational users. Because medical marijuana works and
it works very well, you have to have done the homework in
order to find out what you're looking for and what is going to
help you. Then you have to turn around and experiment on
yourself to try and find the right dosage, the right mix of
cannabinoids that are going to help your system...Recreational
users just use for the high.

Beyond improved health aspects both parties contributed narratives about "the more" of cannabis medicine. "How it helps expand consciousness and extends to all aspects of my life." An Arizona patient shares,

When I started using cannabis on a regular basis, there
became other parts of my life that I wanted to start working
on. It led me down a path of paying more attention to what I

*was putting in my body, my regular habits, even my thought
process, my spiritual process, how I was handling my own
inner things.*

Another shares,

*Cannabis therapy leads you to other things like healthy choices.
The way we eat and how we feel about our bodies.*

Another patient voices, "Cannabis helped me understand there is more than one way to be in the world; there is more than one way of being in this life." A U.S. military veteran and medical cannabis refugee shares,

*My overall quality-of-life has changed. Coming out here and
becoming a patient, starting to use cannabis medicinally, I still
have up and down days, but my overall quality-of-life is 100%
better than it was two or three years ago. It has brought a lot
out inside me. Not just creativity, but being more in depth in
thinking, more involved, especially with my doctors and the
veteran community.*

Chapter Five will include more discussion about the UR and AQAL effects upon it. As well, the following section on Transformative Learning also highlights individual UL experiences.

Transformative Learning

Another objective of this study was to determine if participants engage in *transformative learning* experiences because of engaging in the medical cannabis recommendation process. For the reasons provided in Chapter Three, a transformative learning experience was considered valid if a participant:

✓ reveals a transformed view of themselves;

✓ demonstrates a commitment to help others understand their new perspective; *and*

✓ validates an improvement in communication contributed to the transformation.

Reveals a Transformed View of Themselves

Much as findings in the UL quadrant demonstrate cannabis patients share that they gain a "greater consciousness about myself and others." Physicians shared how they were changed by understanding cannabis medicine, medical cannabis patients, and in a few cases, personal experience using medical cannabis. One Colorado physician shares his own experience with medical cannabis,

> *You can get just so much from listening to patients and their stories. I appreciated it but until I had this severe pain, debilitating pain, where you just are completely consumed with it...When I had it myself, I realized what a remarkable healing herb this is...I saw right away that I personally was experiencing the benefits of medical marijuana.*

Few doctors have this type of experience to share, if they comply with institutionalized zero tolerance drug policies or state compassionate care policies that bar them from using cannabis therapeutically or any other way. A retired Arizona physician conveys how and why he came to recommend medical cannabis,

> *I vowed that if I ever got in a situation where I could offer an alternative to people who were addicted to opioids, alcohol, or cigarettes, that I would do that...[Now], I feel like I am probably helping people more now than I did when I was practicing medicine.*

For all patient participants (20 of 20), the UL awareness was "life-changing." Not only have they found some symptom-relief to aid in recovery, but,

"Being given an opportunity to be someone *besides* a

bed-ridden, chronically ill nobody, changed my life. I am still chronically ill but I am functioning and feeling better about myself."

An exuberant Arizona patient shares,

> I didn't become the typical cannabis advocate. I became the poster child for the legalization of medical cannabis in my state. It changed everything in my life! Since then, I've dedicated my life to this cause.

Another Arizona patient states,

> I started working and helping right after I got my card. I felt like there was a place for me. I had come from a social work background. I saw an opening where I could be in this movement.

Though these stories are strong, for many patients cannabis therapy is simply "about becoming normal again." Being treated as if they were normal is the very challenge they must be strong enough (from an UL perspective) to face.

Demonstrates a Commitment to Help Others Understand Their New Perspective

As shared, most participant stories demonstrate a commitment to help others understand their newly developed perspective. A New Mexico patient and naturopath conveys,

"I believe part of the reason [cannabis therapy

awareness has] been growing is because of people, like me, who spend a lot of time doing community outreach and educating doctors."

An Arizona patient launched a nonprofit as she realized,

When I got my first card, I stopped and thought 'What about the other patients?' So, I formed a patient advocacy organization to help others through the process.

A New Mexico patient shares,

I was very frustrated because it was hard for me to search and find a doctor that would recommend for me. So, I started helping other people. Sending them to cannabis friendly doctors. I became an advocate for the program itself, trying to move it along.

A Colorado patient shares her experience helping other patients,

They [other patients] would ask me questions. I would point them in a direction I thought would help them. Other patients asked me, "How does this help?" and "How do you use it?" [My answers to t]hose questions helped them and they taught somebody else.

A medical cannabis refugee conveys his new perspective,

Cannabis revenue must be used to help society. I have been advocating and working with [NPO] and that gave me a forum. It gave me access to more people. I've seen how the lack of responsibility from the cannabis corporations are causing problems. Therefore, I started bringing awareness and started doing more activism.

Validates an Improvement in Communication Contributed to the Transformation

Paradigmatic shifts in communication are becoming more readily observed in the cannabis community among doctors and patients. As both parties (32 of 32) shared, "Things are getting better out there." Specifically, patient participants recognize that in gaining voice, "I realized that I could be a voice for a lot of different people." A Colorado patient shares how her experience helps other communities of patients,

> *I know there are millions of Lyme disease and Crohn's disease patients out there suffering. We have a better way; they just don't know it! Sharing stories helps people understand.*

An Illinois patient experiencing a full remission from cancer after a terminal diagnosis less than a year prior, shares,

> *As soon as the cannabis changed my life, my wife and I started spending nearly every waking hour of our day educating other people. Our personal lives are ones of complete advocacy and awareness. My wife just looked through stories this morning. We just cannot believe how many success stories we've learned about now. We share these stories every day and hear so many more, it is really incredible.*

Physicians also share stories of patient "enthusiasm and activism" though few (3 of 12) spoke of their own. As noted earlier, it is open communication with patients regarding this subject that helps lead change from within their profession as an advocate, not necessarily from a public activist stance. One doctor shares,

> *It's hard to argue with first-person testimony and sharing my patient's stories really helps others to understand why this has become so important to me. Though it seems out of character*

127

that I am working with marijuana, I am doing it because it
helps my patients.

Another conveys,

I learn from my patients and patients learn from me. I'm
always asking my patients questions because there are more of
them than there are of me. They are saying different things
that aren't even in the research or media yet. This is important
information to learn and share...I pass it on to other doctors
every chance I get.

Chapter Five will discuss these findings in more depth, as well as delve further
into the AQAL findings this chapter explores from participant narrative.

Chapter Five

Findings Discussion

      The purpose of this study is to explore how doctors and patients as participants in compassionate care programs experience the medical cannabis recommendation process. This study seeks to better understand the experiences of doctors and patients as participants in medical cannabis compassionate care programs. It specifically seeks to understand their experiences with the medical cannabis recommendation process. An improved understanding of these experiences viewed through an AQAL framing helps us gain knowledge pertinent to future research in leadership, public policy, healthcare, as well it may have other academic applications. Examining whether system participants experience transformative learning may also provide information relevant to future educational structures.

This chapter will expand upon findings in Chapter Four, as well as discuss additional findings that will direct future research efforts. In this chapter, as in Chapter Four, the narrative findings will be explored following the AQAL frame from the LR quadrants, where the CSA originates and multiplies into additional challenges, to the LL quadrant, societal and cultural impacts from the CSA and related antagonists, to the UR quadrant, for a close view of the doctor-patient relationship, to the UL for an assessment of interior themes from the personal perspective of participants. The chapter will also conclude with an exploration into transformative learning trends discovered within the narrative data.

The following themes were detected early in the data collection process and will be explored in this chapter:

1. The federal CSA has trickledown effect in the LR quadrant to State Public Health Institutions and local medical institution policy. The cumulative effect marginalizes and affects decision-making for system participants across AQAL.

2. Society, and therefore, communities and cultures are transitioning to new social constructs about what it means to use cannabis (LL) and to be a cannabis user (UL). At this critical juncture, public and professional education and social support are necessary, for participants in medical cannabis systems and communities.

3. The doctor-patient relationship is directly and negatively impacted by the CSA, and the LR debris it causes. A frequent and costly side-effect is fragmentation of patient care and disruption of doctor-patient relations (UR).

4. Cultural perceptions (LL) about alternative health care, Holistic Medicine, and substance abuse and addiction seep heavily into myths and taboos about cannabis use.

5. Physicians and patients have both experienced internalized fear, loss of status, stigmatizing judgment, and have been denied personal expression (UL) because of the continued prohibition of cannabis the CSA reinforces.

6. Transformative learning experiences are common within the medical cannabis community, as observed and exhibited in participant stories.

As this study demonstrates, the essence of narrative knowing is to frame and link interactions, like those between doctor and patient, into a plot or storyline. From asking questions like, "Can you tell me how you came to recommend (physician) or request to be recommended (patient) medical cannabis?" participants could provide storied responses based on their experience and perception of the situation. Integral theory provides a structure from which these interactions or experiences may be understood. Utilizing collective narratives and the AQAL frame helps link individual events (UR) to the larger whole (AQAL). Throughout this project, the AQAL frame structured participant narratives so that a clear *big-picture* is revealed. This kind of knowledge provides a rich, resonant comprehension of a person's situation as it unfolds in time. It also helps develop a clear understanding of the factors one must consider (and may experience) if requesting or proffering a medical cannabis recommendation, which is the study's objective.

Unlike scientific knowledge, through which a detached and replaceable observer generates or comprehends replicable and generalizable information, narrative knowledge leads to particular understanding about a specific situation by a participant, or in this case a group of participants (Bruner, 1986, p. 18-19). Life story is localized in the UL quadrant, but interpretation is influenced by UR and LL relational and cultural perspectives, as well as LR social situations. Though physicians and patients have different interests in the conversation regarding medical cannabis recommendation (UR), both appear to experience many of the same concerns (AQAL), though personal perspectives differ, to some degree, based on the role in the relationship, as narrative throughout Chapter Four demonstrates.

LR: Institutions, Systems, and Processes

State compassionate care policies have been a primary focus of advocacy groups related to patient access for "safe, legal" cannabis medication that is "taxed and regulated," as noted in Chapter One. These policies and the resulting programs, fall squarely within the LR quadrant, as does the federal CSA; yet, the conflict between federal and state bleeds over into AQAL. As participant testimony suggests, current medical cannabis policies do not answer Rawls' call for justice-as-fairness (Schwartz, 2013, p 271). There can be no justice, when state policies directly conflict with federal ones.

During this study, the U.S. government acted upon this issue in a manner that was described as "despicable" and "asinine" by participants. In response to a 2011 petition, urging the D.E.A. to reclassify cannabis as a drug with accepted medical use. The D.E.A. refused to reclassify cannabis; however, action was taken to "relax certain restrictions for growing marijuana for research purposes" (Reuters, August 11, 2016). "An extremely small victory." For physicians and patients participating in this study, this outcome was "meaningless." As one patient conveys, "The situation remains the same, we're all still federal criminals."

The federal restrictions against *cannabis sativa* are certainly the greatest obstacle for physicians and patients, as demonstrated in Chapter Four narrative findings. More than half of the States and the District of Columbia have policies that stand in direct opposition to the CSA. However, as discussed in Chapter Two, the consequences for medical cannabis patients are still steep under state policies that conflict directly with the federal CSA. Both physicians and patients have justifiable fears when considering whether they will oppose federal drug policy and engage in a state medical cannabis program. These conflicts impact our social systems and every single person who seeks assistance or needs support from them. The D.E.A. interference described by physicians and patients in Chapter Four is common. Intimidation is a powerful tool and has successfully maintained social control in this arena for nearly 80 years.

Political Power-as-Dominance: D.E.A. Interference

"Is this legal?" was the first question participants asked themselves when initially faced with a request for or a thought of requesting their own medical cannabis recommendation. The answer is confusing. Within some state's borders a registered cannabis patient has specific rights granted, as well physicians have certain protections granted. However, on the federal level, patients have no right to use cannabis medicinally, but the physicians' protections are assured, as they have been successfully challenged in courts of law.

The 2003 finding in *Walters vs. Conant* from a California Federal District Court decided that it is the right of a doctor to discuss the use of cannabis with patients and to issue a written or oral recommendation to use cannabis without fear of legal reprisal. Many of the participating physicians (5 of 12) "stumbled upon this case" through personal research and discussed it during interviews. As one relays:

> *Was this even something I could do legally as a physician? Finding the court case from 2003 ...where doctors were being sued or charged by the D.E.A. for distributing marijuana for signing recommendations in California. Basically, it was decided that it was the right of the doctor to sign these recommendations... practicing cannabis medicine is based on First Amendment rights. The doctor is not providing the illegal substance, but just talking about it must be protected. Not only for a doctor to pursue a livelihood, which is essentially what it is for, but even more importantly for a patient to have Freedom of Speech ... So, I knew that the D.E.A. - that I was not going to be - I'm not going to be charged with something, just for doing that...that made it, in my mind,* do-able.'

Because of the phenomenal disengagement between federal and state drug policies, no party to any medical cannabis program system is acting fully within the law, if they possess, consume, cultivate, or purchase cannabis. During these times, they are in violation of federal statutes per the CSA and corresponding D.E.A regulations. Under LR "Additional Findings" several patient stories regarding state-level interference with patients and caregivers in "seemingly medical or legal" states are examined further.

Physician and patient participants both share stories of D.E.A. interference throughout the medical cannabis community. Specifically, federal agents "harass and intimidate" physicians "who step outside conventional health care organizations." For doctors, practicing Integrative Cannabis and offering recommendation evaluation services almost exclusively, this type of harassment is "experienced frequently - at least, several times per year."

> "The void we [physicians] fill is real and more support is critically needed...but you have to be ready to stand up to authority."

Patient participants agree, "Who are you supposed to go to when all of your doctors work for the same medical system and aren't allowed to recommend medical cannabis?"

Large medical institutions frequently have policies in place restricting physicians from recommending medical cannabis to patients to avoid the threat of D.E.A. interference, at least in part. Some institutional policies make exceptions for patients with certain qualifying medical conditions, usually terminal cancer, but many do not. These institutional policies force most patients seeking a recommendation to go outside personal healthcare systems and away from provided insurance coverage (LR), as well as his or her primary and specialty care physicians (UR). The result is; not only additional out-of-pocket expenses for the patient to incur (UL/UR), but a fragmentation of the patient's care (UR/LL/LR), a loss of support (UL/UR/LL), and an interior reinforcement of the dominant narrative (UL). "Having to go to a pot doctor makes me feel like this is not legitimately legal." Yet, as participants agree, "Until the D.E.A. changes the Schedule I status, we are all still criminals to some degree and the system treats us as such. It really does." D.E.A. interference in health decisions is a prime example of the structural violence associated with cannabis that threatens physicians who recommend medical cannabis - and the patients who are registered to use it.

Law, which comes from policies like the CSA, can be a means of preventing or resolving the enactment of stigma as violence, discrimination, or other harm or it can be an avenue through which stigma is created or reinforced. For nearly 80 years, cannabis laws have been a means of violence against citizens. Changing the social constructs (LL) is perhaps more challenging than changing the laws (LR). For a patient with a chronic or terminal health condition, who is dually stigmatized (UL/LL) as a registered cannabis patient, acceptance of society's views (LL) and self-stigmatization (UL) lead to concealment (UR) to avoid discrimination. Considering, medical conditions vary dramatically in the extent to which they are socially significant. Compare hypertension, bone fractures, and melanoma, for example, with incontinence, AIDS, and schizophrenia. Then add cannabis use for "a double-whammy." However, concealment itself is plagued by lifelong hidden distress and unhappiness (UL) experienced by those who *conceal*. "Hiding it made me feel like a criminal, even though I was using it legally, I wasn't using it freely."

Again, as described in Chapter Four findings, D.E.A. interference in healthcare decisions is a prime example of structural violence associated with medical cannabis. The CSA classifies *cannabis sativa* as a Schedule I drug with a "high potential for abuse" and "no accepted medical use," in the same schedule as drugs such as heroin, LSD, and ecstasy. Meanwhile, oxycodone and methadone, the most commonly abused prescription drugs and leading sources of opioid overdose deaths, are Schedule II drugs; implying that these drugs are less dangerous than cannabis though unlike opioids, it cannot induce a fatal overdose in and of itself. Per the Centers for Disease Control,

> "As many as 1 in 4 people who receive prescription opioids - long term for noncancer pain in primary care settings - *struggle with addiction*."

(CDC.gov). Recent reports show that in 2014, "47,055 American citizens died from drug overdoses - 1.5 times greater than the number killed in car crashes" (Kounang, December 18, 2015). *Cannabis sativa* is non-toxic, responsible for zero deaths by overdose, thereby making its CSA classification seem unjustified (Nelson, 2015), as discussed in Chapter One.

Arguably cannabis is improperly classified in the Schedule I category. In contrast, cannabis patients and healthcare providers stand on the conviction that cannabis may in fact be closer in relation to herbal therapies such as St. John's Wort (Nelson, 2014). St. John's Wort is not regulated by the Controlled Substances Act; instead it is an over-the-counter (OTC) medication with labeling that attests it is only a dietary supplement *and* has no confirmed medicinal value. Perhaps the removal of cannabis (or its combined family of cannabinoids) from the CSA is unachievable for now, as it runs counter to dominant notions that demonize this plant-based medication. However, whole-plant remedies like "Rick Simpson Oil" (essential oil distilled from the *cannabis sativa* plant) are being used widely and successfully, as attested to by patient participants (16 of 20) for a wide variety of treatments, suggesting not only that a Schedule I classification is unwarranted, but also that FDA approval is unnecessary for cannabis in whole-plant forms.

During his 2008 campaign, President Obama committed to ending federal cannabis raids, which frequently target registered cannabis patients, particularly if they grow cannabis. Asset forfeiture is included among the options federal, state, county or city agents may take. In a press release President Obama stated, "I will not have the Justice Department prosecuting and raiding medical marijuana users. It's not a good use of our resources (Chester, VA, 2008)." Statements such as this are welcome in the medical cannabis community. In fact, shortly after Obama took office, the Department of Justice (DOJ) issued the "Ogden memo," which directed U.S. Attorneys not to target medical marijuana providers "whose actions are in clear compliance with existing state laws," producing a sigh of relief in the medical cannabis community that led to expansion of patient services significantly increasing the number of medical cannabis businesses (Freedom is Green). This reprieve was short-lived, even though more states began implementing medical cannabis policies and programs in response to public outcries for relief. However, the "Cole memo" issued in June 2011, took an incongruent position, informing U.S. Attorneys that they may target medical cannabis providers whether or not they comply with state laws. This memo stands in opposition to statements both President Obama and former Attorney General Eric Holder made public. The Ogden Memorandum was "never intended to shield such activities from federal enforcement action and prosecution, even where those activities purport to comply with state law" (Cole Memo). As participants attest, particularly patient participants, "No one is really sure if it's safe to be a patient or not. We hear of people getting busted all the time for doing just what I am doing. It's not just the feds, these state police love cooperating for the asset money." The CSA is stuck in the status quo and neither scientists nor advocates have found the momentum or political support to shift this incredibly dense federal obstacle from the path. The following section explores the LR trickledown effects of the CSA Schedule I restriction demonstrated earlier in Chapter Four.

Additional LR Research Findings

One of the greatest problems with the federal D.E.A. interference is that it flows down to state and local law enforcement.

"Society cannot allow a drug enforcement agency to come between doctors and patients."

Though issues in this area were not broached by participating physicians (0 of 12), all patient participants (20 of 20) commented about "extra-legal" consequences of using cannabis, as well as mentioning that the status of *medical cannabis patient* does little to deflect discrimination, fear, stigmatizing experiences, or "lower the fear of retaliatory behavior from those in authority who oppose my newfound rights." For patients new to cannabis therapy and considering the possible consequences of requesting a recommendation, having an available state program may make it appear legal for a registered patient to possess or consume cannabis, but it seems a staggering number of patients have found "medical cannabis is not really legal because of the Schedule I status" and places them in danger of criminal prosecution or asset forfeiture. Stories like these affect others and it is difficult to assure patients that registering as a medical cannabis patient is legal, "when after we do, we find out that it really isn't."

Shockingly, nearly a third of participating patients (6 of 20) share experiences of interference by police ranging from D.U.I. (Driving Under the Influence) stops, criminal charges (frequently dropped later), or fines. Patients share stories of:
- ✓ Five vehicles searched
- ✓ Two stops resulting in charges of D.U.I., both cases pending

- ✓ Two non-D.U.I. fines imposed
- ✓ Three vehicles towed

Additionally, two patients have received fines for public marijuana use. In his account, a participating patient was found guilty of misdemeanor possession and public intoxication and fined $500 for using cannabis in his own garage after a neighbor smelled it and reported it to police. That he had a legal right to consume cannabis on his own property never entered the defense, his patient status was excluded from his legal defense. Like other patients, he finds his rights as a medical cannabis patient do not always extend to a defense in court, even though the state had sanctioned his actions by registering him as a medical cannabis patient.

In addition to the above stories, a significant 10% (2 of 20) of patients participating in this study are or may be under asset forfeiture. Asset forfeiture occurs when local and/or state law enforcement interact (with or without federal support) to seize a patient's property. The person is never charged with a crime. Administrative forfeiture is the process by which property may be seized and forfeited in the United States *without* judicial involvement. The authority for a seizing agency to start an administrative forfeiture action is found in 19 U.S.C. § 1607 which states, "Civil forfeiture is a proceeding brought against the property rather than against the person who committed the offense. Civil forfeiture does not require either criminal charges against the owner of the property or a criminal conviction." In other words, if law enforcement suspects a person(s) is in violation of federal or state drug laws they may seize their property without ever charging the person with an actual crime.

During interviews for this study (August 2016), two (2) participating Colorado patients were aggressively searched and more than $20,000 in personal possessions have been seized. To date (March 3, 2017), no charges have been filed, nor have the patient-caregivers even been questioned by the Colorado city police department who has seized their property. The participant's attorney "suspects that their assets will be seized by local law enforcement under federal or state asset forfeiture regulations" since this is still common practice in Colorado.

Another 10% of patient participants already have experienced asset forfeiture, though this was unknown to the researcher prior to the interviews. This means that 20%

(4 of 20) of this study's participants may have lost more than $300,000 in property by participant estimates (vehicles, safes, jewelry, cash, cannabis, and other items) to asset seizure, in the past two years (2014-2016, in either Colorado or California). This data surprised the researcher and is an appalling finding that requires further exploration outside of this study.

It is horrifying to find that 20% of this small study's patient participants have been harmed by using the small measure of rights they received with the status of registered medical cannabis patient.

"These outcomes are not the intent the voters of this state had in mind when they thought they legalized medical cannabis."

The harassment of cannabis patients by law enforcement seldom makes local, much less national news, nor are criminal charges filed in many of the cases (particularly, if assets have been seized); however, stories like the following are common. Stories like these are rampant enough that "fear that it might happen to me" causes duress for many patients and stops others from pursuing cannabis as a viable therapy option. The following story is a familiar example,

> [An Illinois cannabis patient has been pulled over for speeding; 65-mph in a 55-mph zone; his medical cannabis registry is connected to his driver's license record]. The officer went back to his vehicle and sat there for ten or fifteen minutes. He comes back and says, 'I have a canine in route toward your vehicle. Is he going to hit on anything when he gets here?' 'Oh, I don't imagine he will hit on anything illegal but I do have my medical bag in the back.' 'Your medical bag?' I said, 'Yes, I have medical cannabis in there and I have my medical cannabis card right here.' I hand him my medical card... I stepped out of

the van and opened the sliding back door, pulled out the medical bag and hand it to him. He said, 'Have a seat back in your vehicle.' So, I had a seat back in my vehicle. I watch him go to his car and dump my bag all over the hood of his cruiser. He fumbles around with things that he can't open - everything is child-proof - and finally throws everything back in the bag and comes back to my car. He gets me and my daughter, my six-year old daughter, out of the van. I was taking her to VBS (vacation bible school). He brought us back to his cruiser and put her in the back seat and put me in the front seat. He threw my bag in the trunk. I turned toward him, my daughter is in the backseat looking at me horrified and I said, 'It's alright sweetie, it's okay, you didn't do anything.' I ask him, 'Am I under arrest or am I being charged with something?' He goes, 'We'll figure that out here in a little bit.' [The police office allows the patient to call his wife, she leaves work to drive frantically to the side of the road to pick up their daughter]. After she leaves with our daughter, I ask again, 'Am I under arrest or being charged with something?' He said, 'I am going to have your vehicle towed.' I said, 'For what reason?' He says, 'You're getting charged for what you have in that bag.' I said, 'You have my medical cannabis card. I handed that to you just a minute ago, I am good to have that. That's my medicine.' He goes, 'Well, we'll figure out what the charges are when we get to the jail.'

The patient was held without bond for nearly 36 hours before he was released with a "summons to appear in court about 5 weeks later."

The withdrawal effects of pharmaceuticals he was denied while in custody exacerbated his illness significantly; he required time off work and a reduced work schedule for several months following this incident. Further, it was weeks after (when the patient showed up to his court date with an attorney, he'd been forced to retain) to

140

find no charges had ever been filed. A probable minor traffic violation - he never received a speeding ticket though he was stopped for exceeding posted speed limits - turned into a $2,000 nightmare (tow bill, lost work, attorney retainer, and his medical cannabis medication was not returned to him though it was seized in licensed dispensary packaging) accompanied by significant health issues that continue to be problematic for the patient on a day-to-day basis.

The 40-year old white male patient observes, "If I had been a minority, I'd have died in that cell from withdrawal. It doesn't matter that I was within the law now, that would have made it worse." While stories like this may appear to be outside the doctor-patient relationship, this experience will flow into it and beyond, into AQAL of the person affected and those he shares his story with. "Imagining this type of treatment may exist, conquering the fears that it won't, and then having it happen, that changes a person. It makes you realize you are just an unwilling participant in the war on drugs."

Federal Border Patrol

Further concern for medical cannabis patients living in a southern U.S. state is the ever-present Border Patrol. Five (5 of 8) patient participants living within these states breached the subject of Border Patrol while sharing his or her story. States like California, Arizona, and New Mexico either directly border or are within security boundaries of the U.S. Border Patrol in relation to the Mexico border. California has had a medical cannabis program since 1996, New Mexico, 2007 and Arizona, 2010, yet 25% of participating patients (5 of 32) or 62% that are registered cannabis patients living in these a border states (5 of 8), either self-reported an incident or provided details of incidents that happened to other patients within the state's borders. These stories highlight the importance of resolving this issue federally and demonstrate how UL/UR/LL quadrants are affected by LR policies. A New Mexico physician declares,

> *Well, it is federally illegal. They aren't doing it as much now as they were doing it before, they have eased up. Before they would arrest you, even if you were a cannabis patient. They'd hassle you. Now what the patients tell me is that "They took my*

medicine. They made me throw it away!" This happens! It's horrible! It is just horrible for the patient!

An Arizona physician proclaims,

When you have a cancer patient that just went to a dispensary and bought some tincture, chocolates, and some salve. They've spent hundreds of dollars. Then they go through a checkpoint and the dogs alert. They take the patient's medicine away from them!

A California patient shares his frightening and marginalizing experience,

My son and I were near San Diego...when we got stopped at a checkpoint by border patrol. Now, mind you, we had not been to Mexico, we'd been to a dispensary and were less than 20 minutes from our home. Also, we are both natural-born American citizens and both have a medical marijuana license. When they asked if the dogs would hit on anything, I told them "They won't hit on anything illegal, but I have my medical marijuana and my license in that bag," as I pointed to the backseat and my locked bag. They ransacked both of us, individually, and my vehicle and everything in it. I didn't get a ticket or anything, but they took $400 in cannabis - along with the dispensary receipt, $300 plus in cash from our wallets, and walked away - just drove off without another word, like thieves. It would cost me in more in attorney fees than $700, so they won. They robbed me and there is nothing I can do about it. No one I can report it to that will help. It is still very traumatizing to think about that day.

Though these patients live in a state that supports a medical cannabis program, the Schedule I status of *cannabis sativa* federally continues to interfere with hard-won rights.

There is a huge disconnect between the Schedule I status and how patients are healing with this plant. The Border Patrol ignores state law and harasses patients because they can. They're federal, they can.

Though both patients and physicians have the right to engage in a conversation about the recommendation and use of cannabis, if it remains a Schedule I substance, they will continue to expect and fear federal interference and intimidation.

Knowledge Control: Research Hindered

Although little federal or state funding is made available for projects that consider the medical efficacy of a Schedule I substance in humans, this same lack of research is frequently offered as a valid reason for rejecting medical cannabis programs by the D.E.A. itself, as well as Senators, Congressmen, Governors, state-appointed medical cannabis boards, institutions, insurance companies, and voters.

"The lawmakers say we don't have human trials, but they have hundreds of people standing on the Capitol steps who know that cannabis heals. Yet, no one will research us."

Schedule I status has an immensely negative impact on research because it has indefinitely stalled the medical establishment's preferred human trial model, the randomized clinical trial (RCT). Despite having more than two million medical cannabis patients registered across the U.S., the number of human trials and studies related to any medical application for cannabis can be counted on your fingers. They are few and far between. This failure is directly tied to the Schedule I status as a participating physician describes,

143

We are decades behind because of the drug war and prohibition. I'm glad to hear that it sounds like N.I.D.A. and D.E.A. are going to loosen up restrictions for research. That's great but it still continues the drug war. It still means that a whole lot of patients are left waiting for the research when they could be using this great plant and getting relief.

This rather optimistic statement was dashed just a few days following this physician's interview when the D.E.A. announced (Reuters, August 11, 2016) it would not be reclassifying *cannabis sativa*. As mentioned earlier, there can be no *justice*, when state policies directly conflict with federal ones. When the D.E.A. refused to reclassify cannabis in August, authorities simply reinforced, the stigma and marginalization attached to the use of cannabis.

As participants note, there are "thousands of studies on cannabis, the endocannabinoid system, and lots of animal studies. The only thing we're lacking is collecting all this data that patients are walking around with." Physicians participating in this study agree, "With proper funding there are thousands of good community-based trials just here in this city, expand that around the nation and we could quickly learn a lot more about this."

The NIDA and NIH have begun investing in cannabis research, primarily by funding eCS and synthetic cannabinoid research outside the U.S. In fact, they invested approximately $9 million to fund fifteen (15) cannabis related research projects in 2015 (report.nida.gov). NIDA research represents a small portion of the NIH $30.9 billion annual budget at only $1.05 billion. However, the cannabis research budget represents less than 1% of NIDA's budget. Human trials are not a focus and though the D.E.A. has "relaxed certain restrictions for growing marijuana for research purposes," it's doubtful that "the floodgates to randomized controlled trials will be opened" by "this miniscule change in restrictions," shares another participating physician.

As mentioned in Chapter Four, given the D.E.A. interference, both physicians and patients are resigned that,

[Until rescheduling Cannabis] "There aren't going to be any human studies done. We can't do those now because of the Schedule I status."

In other words, it is going to be some time before patients and physicians can answer the questions "How is this going to work for my condition?" or "How will this help my patient?"

State Compassionate Care Policies

State medical cannabis public policies fall squarely within the LR quadrant and have been a primary focus of advocacy groups related to patient access for "safe, legal" cannabis medication that is "taxed and regulated" outside the federal CSA system. This study finds, *justice as fairness* is not at play in medical cannabis policies. Often patients experience (18 of 20), "our state's administration is unfriendly with the medical cannabis industry and patients" and physicians support this belief (9 of 12).

Medical cannabis compassionate care policies have both social benefits and social harms intrinsically imposed within them. The social harms are directly related to the Schedule I status of *cannabis sativa*. The greatest social benefit is gaining access to cannabis legally and having a small modicum of rights established as a registered medical cannabis patient *within* the state you reside. Prior to requesting a recommendation for medical cannabis from his or her physician or "spending the money for a marijuana doctor," patients typically engage with the State Department of Public Health. As patients (12 of 12) share in Chapter Four, navigating a new state program was "worth it in the end, because it represents less suffering than I had before," but as was revealed, the newfound rights (LR) came with an AQAL sacrifice, as the following sections explore in more detail.

Public Health Initiatives: Public Health Departments

State medical cannabis public policies fall squarely within the LR quadrant and have been a primary focus of ballot initiatives and advocacy groups though most patients find them to be rather "frosty with the medical cannabis industry and patients." The vast number of medical cannabis program failings brought up by participants cannot be adequately discussed within this study. Reviewing a few critical areas will help direct future research related to the administration of these programs by Public Health Departments. It would also help readers understand how these systems affect participant decision-making and may discourage chronically and terminally ill people from seeking a recommendation for medical cannabis.

From a policy and regulation perspective, for patients navigating a state medical cannabis program's application and registry process, obtaining a medical cannabis recommendation from a physician is the first course of action after making "the decision to apply." Research that aids in this decision is frequently accessed via a State Public Health Department website. Like other government websites (i.e. healthcare.gov), these tend to be far from user-friendly. As one Illinois patient shares,

> "I immediately got on their webpage and started the application process...that turned into a two-day excursion."

Even for those with computer experience, as patient participant stories demonstrate, the process "can be quite difficult" and requires "patience and persistence." Further, few of these websites provide patients or physicians with *accurate* information regarding cannabis, dosing instructions, or other pertinent information that may be necessary for an informed decision about the subject.

Additionally, for physicians they often fail to provide more than the required recommendation form the doctor is to complete. Seldom, do health departments provide guidelines or instructions beyond how to complete the form correctly. As stated in Chapter Four, both parties believe, "There needs to be a strategic plan put into place about how this is going to be regulated and how people are going to be educated and informed about it." Typically, public health plans trickle down from the federal government to the states; in this case, "the system is broken uniquely in each new medical cannabis program."

Unlike many state-funded programs, medical cannabis programs are usually financially fluid due to the influx of patient and industry fees they receive. Failing to offer physician or public education or accurate information about the program, participant responsibilities, or the use of cannabis medications negatively impacts both parties. This predicament leaves participants wondering, "If, perhaps, more doctors were given this information, more would provide recommendations for patients?"

Participant suggestions of instructional guides, "factual public service announcements," continuing medical education courses, and other "public health support that is given to normal health programs" would go a long way to remedying Health Department communication regarding designated medical cannabis programs. This information will be discussed further in the section on Education (LL).

Recently (April 2, 2015), the Colorado Department of Public Health (CDPH) issued guidelines for physicians recommending medical cannabis. The participating Colorado physicians noted that they support these guidelines. As well, they acknowledge that these guidelines were "hard won" after attempts by the Colorado Department of Public Health to "destroy the medical marijuana program." After all,

"If no doctors will perform recommendations, then there won't be any new patients. The dispensaries will go out of business and this whole matter will just go away. Right?"

However, the CDPH policy is written clearly as one that establishes "the criteria for referring physicians to the Department of Regulatory Agencies (DORA) Medical Board for Investigation." It would better serve as a deterrent rather than a recruitment tool for physicians. In other words,

> *If you don't follow these guidelines you will be punished, much like those four doctors that have recently been suspended. They pushed too hard on plant counts for patients or had too many patients. Whatever the reason, the state wanted them to slow down or stop and they didn't conform, so their punishment is at the very least public humiliation and possibly the loss of their livelihood.*

This Colorado physician was referring to the recent suspension of four (4) Colorado physicians by DORA that has been publicized across Colorado news media as a "warning shot from the state to comply or else lose your license" (Ingold, 2016). This is but one example that demonstrates that medical cannabis policies have both social benefits and social harms intrinsically imposed within them for all participants in the new system.

Perhaps one of the biggest obstacles to operating the state-level medical cannabis programs is the fact that they are outside the norm for Health Departments. As one Colorado patient attests,

"I don't know any other medicine that you must apply to the state for and pay money to go to a special doctor, who doesn't even know you, so you can get a license to use it. Not any other. In and of itself, this program is set up to be discriminatory to our state's suffering citizens."

Programs being set-up for failure is not unheard of, and suggesting that medical cannabis programs are "purposefully designed to fail those they are meant to serve" is a consensus opinion of patient (20 of 20) and physician (6 of 12) participants, based on the stories they shared during interviews.

Insurance Complications

In the United States, the clear majority of physicians are connected to or directly employed by hospital and clinic systems, which ties them all directly to federal funding through programs like Medicaid and Medicare, and Veterans Administration benefits, as discussed in Chapters One and Four. Budget conscious administrators afraid of funding loss implement policies meant to protect the organization and assure that the institution is complying with federal CSA. However, in taking these policy actions, they fail to recognize that every single patient and practitioner is negatively impacted (AQAL) by the federal government's inability to recognize the public health implications of this LR issue.

As participating patients experienced, it is commonplace for healthcare organizations to enact policies (LR) that bar physicians from engaging in the recommendation process. Having medical cannabis recommendations managed outside a patient's normal healthcare system (LR) means the treatment can quickly, if not already, be cost prohibitive (UL) for the majority (LL). Other institutes place obstacles in the path of physicians seeking to recommend medical cannabis to patients. An Illinois doctor shares,

> *I was required to take an online course regarding substance abuse before I could request to be allowed to recommend cannabis. The class was online but it was four hours long, a lot of time out of my day. The worse part was that in the entire course the subject of cannabis, even as a substance of abuse, never came up. It was never mentioned. It was just a hoop to jump through. The first hoop they threw me.*

The lack of attention to this issue solidifies a black market because it places legal access at a point of unaffordability or is too cumbersome for those who could most benefit from it. The newly launched medical cannabis pilot program in Illinois is among the first to require a "bona fide" doctor-patient relationship as a condition of approval for the program. In other words, evaluation centers, sometimes referred to as "pot doctors" are not allowed. Neither are legitimate Integrative Cannabis practices. This leaves patients scrambling for support as witnessed by approximately 9,000 currently registered patients (Wright, 05/15/16). Although I have been a registered medical cannabis patient in three other states and have extensive medical records validating three of Illinois' "qualifying conditions," in a year's time I could not obtain a medical cannabis recommendation through my normal healthcare channels.

While the Illinois Department of Public Health has been tasked with managing a medical cannabis program, they failed to set parameters on what constitutes a "bona fide" doctor-patient relationship. Though the instituted regulations require a bona fide relationship, beyond vaguely describing non-evaluation center relationships (e.g. ongoing, accepts insurance, attachment to a recognized clinic or hospital), neither patients or physicians fully understand what this requirement means initially. For patients, it eventually means having to spend $600-$750 for three or more appointments, with a physician outside his or her normal health care system, to establish a bona-fide or *recurring* relationship.

In contrast, patients in California also require an evaluation service, in most cases, but the cost is $40-$60 per year for one visit because any doctor may recommend medical cannabis, if allowed by his or her medical institution. Further, physicians filling these roles have been threatened by the Illinois Department of Health, much as Colorado physicians are under attack for over-prescribing medical cannabis plant counts (Ingold, July 19, 2016). Already more patients have been denied from primary or specialty physicians than have been approved (IDPH Report, June 2015). Of those noted in the IDPH June 2015 Report as probable "work-around" patients, over 1,500 and perhaps as many as 2,500 approved medical cannabis patients, represents between $900,000-$1,500,000 out of the pockets of terminally and chronically ill patients; payment for a recommendation outside the bona-fide doctor-patient relationship. Given the political climate it's not hard to understand why both parties are concerned. As a Washington physician states, "The Illinois story isn't good because we needed this outside system so long as doctors on the inside didn't do it. They still don't. It's kind of necessary."

As discussed by physician participants in Chapter Four, for recommending doctors, insurance requirements extend beyond the companies they regularly rely on and deal with (for patient benefits and service payments to medical malpractice and other business liability requirements they must meet to practice medicine). As one Colorado physician shares, she "felt the pressure and intimidation" in these institutional actions. "I mean if your insurance company says, 'don't do it', you don't do it." Each of these institutions have established independent policies and practices (LR), meaning it is often difficult for doctors to find support should they decide to work with medical cannabis patients and submit medical cannabis recommendations to the state. The LR policies of insurance companies "play a prominent role in decision-making" for physicians considering whether they should proffer a medical cannabis recommendation to a requesting patient and are a result of the continued Schedule I status of cannabis.

Public Health Departments

Examples of harms to patients that participate in medical cannabis programs plagued patient participant stories. Since the researcher verified that every patient was currently registered within his or her state of residence, several patient participants (11 of 20) took an opportunity to comment on the state's certification or renewal process. None of the comments were favorable and the majority convey that "the Health Department definitely scares people off from applying. If I hadn't been sure this was an option I wanted to take, if I didn't know better, then the people and the process would have scared me off too."

Additionally, all four (4 of 32) participants from the State of New Mexico shared issues with the Public Health Department's lack of response,

"I called every day for three weeks straight and went

right to voicemail. Every day I left my phone number and a detailed message. I finally went down there and stood in front of someone so I could be served. I was so frustrated."

and delays, "The State of New Mexico is running 90 to 120 days late, so people's cards are expiring". Verifying the Health Department delays in the State of New Mexico, one patient participant's medical card was expired at the time we first scheduled an interview. He eventually received his medical cannabis card and was able to participate in the study. However, the patient had not had access to a dispensary in more than three (3) months and was in violation of New Mexico marijuana laws during that time. Possessing and using his medication without a current registration exposes him to criminal penalties. Although several of the above testimonies discuss New Mexico's Public Health Department delays, patients in each state shared similar problematic issues. These issues do not seem to be unique to only one state's program, but rather are products of poor state policy that conflict with federal policies.

During the summer of 2016, the New Mexico Health Department delays made statewide news (Lopez, 2016) and the response of the program director was a "typical" example of what system participants have "come to expect." Confirming participant concerns, Department of Health, Medical Cannabis Program Director, Kenny Vigil suggested,

> *I think that our message to patients whose card isn't up to date*
> *at this time; they should really contact their medical provider*
> *to see if they can find some other type of relief until they can get*
> *their card (Teague, 2016).*

As the program requires, all registered patients have already *exhausted* conventional treatments prior to applying to the medical cannabis program.

A majority now rely on cannabis in conjunction with conventional therapies or as a replacement for pharmaceutical treatments. For patients and physicians within the State of New Mexico this response from the State Health Department was unacceptable and demonstrates the obstacles they face from the program administration. As a New Mexico physician conveys, "After weaning pharmaceuticals, it is horrific to lose the medicine that *does* work, but being told to go back to how you felt before by the program's Director is unacceptable and just plain wrong."

State Health Departments have a regretful reputation with medical cannabis patients because of bureaucratic habits that are deeply ingrained. Three patient participants (3 of 20) reported "breaches of confidentiality" by Health Departments in three different states. Each of these cases involved the Health Department either sending the participant information meant for another patient or having another patient contact the participant because they'd received information meant for the participant. An Illinois patient shares,

> *Some guy calls me because my phone number was on the*
> *paperwork he received. He says, 'I have your stuff. I thought it*
> *was mine when I opened it. Did you happen to get my stuff?'*
> *No, I did not get his paperwork, but he sure had mine.*

Though these issues are outside the scope of this study, these critical breaches of confidentiality should be explored further.

Another side of the insurance company-doctor relationship also involves pharmaceutical companies and medications that are "covered by these plans and for which doctors are paid to prescribe," sometimes. Patient participants (20 of 20), unlike, physician participants (0 of 12), discuss the relationships doctors, insurance companies (and/or pharmaceutical companies) have and did so in negative terms. Expressing frustration, a Connecticut patient voices,

> *They should stop caring about writing prescriptions. They are*
> *being paid to write prescriptions. As well, insurance companies*
> *offer them [physicians] more money to write prescriptions for*
> *"this drug or this brand." They need to care more about how*
> *the cannabis is helping a patient than how many prescriptions*

they write and refill.

A patient in Illinois expresses,

> *He can give me something he knows can kill me or he can*
> *support what I am doing that is non-toxic and helpful. He'd*
> *prefer to write the dangerous prescription because that's what*
> *he knows to do and because the pharmaceutical company will*
> *send him on a fishing trip. It's just wrong.*

A Colorado patient shares the following experience,

> *My doctor ran down the hall and put a prescription in my hand*
> *that we'd just discussed would make my symptoms worse - and*
> *I was already dying! She said, "Maybe you want to use more*
> *cannabis to help control the side-effects but I think you should*
> *at least fill this prescription?" Was she getting a kick-back on*
> *that script? If not, why was she pushing it at me?*

Are patients justified in these beliefs? Studies suggest they are (Dalta & Dalta, 2016; Scheurich, 2014); as well, ProPublica began tracking pharmaceutical company payments to doctors in 2010 (www.DollarsforDocs.com), as a public service. Per ProPublica 2016 findings

"The more physicians learn about a new drug's 'differentiating characteristics' the more likely they are to prescribe it. The more they prescribe it, the more likely they are to be selected as speakers or consultants for the company or receive other financial benefits."

As a non-pharmaceutical and Schedule I Controlled Substance, no such support exists for cannabis and this is a point of frustration for patients (20 of 20).

Healthcare benefits are not the only insurance issue medical cannabis patients face. As described by six patient participants (6 of 20), the medical cannabis patient status has interfered with life insurance and disability insurance benefits. An Illinois patient shares,

> My life insurance company denied me because I smoke marijuana. I had admitted that to one of my doctors many years ago and they found it in my records. You have to be seven years "free of marijuana" before they'll allow you to buy more life insurance. "It's only been four according to your records." That's the last time I openly admitted I use to a doctor. I'm still with the same doctor so I assume he knows I still do.

A patient in California receiving SSI disability benefits conveys,

> I am afraid I will lose my disability benefits if they find out that I've weaned 95% of the pharmaceuticals. I am still disabled, but my quality-of-life is much better. I don't think the disability claims adjuster will care about my quality-of-life.

There is progress. In 2015, New Mexico became the first state to support medical cannabis as a covered or reimbursable benefit for workman's compensation injuries. The New Mexico Workmen's Compensation Association's process requires insurance carriers to reimburse the injured workers (who are registered medical cannabis patients) directly for medical marijuana costs, a first for medical cannabis patients nationwide (O'Catherine, 2015).

Institutional Policies

Historically, hospitals and clinics institute medical cannabis policies prohibiting attending or resident physicians or those associated with the healthcare systems from recommending cannabis shortly after medical cannabis programs are launched. All already have zero tolerance drug policies in place, to satisfy federal contracts that require they comply with the CSA. Even in California, where cannabis has been medicalized since 1996, a patient shares,

> *My primary care doctor still can't recommend for me, even though I've been her patient and a cannabis patient for more than six years. She knows it helps me and would be happy to do it, but the system won't allow her to. So, I see her for some things and my medical cannabis doctor specifically, for a recommendation each year. That's just the way it is...it's what I have to do.*

Participating patients (15 of 20) seeking a recommendation "believe most institutions have already implemented these policies, so many don't even inquire." For physicians, open to recommending cannabis therapy "a closed institutional door is frequently enough to change their mind. No doctor wants to take on an issue like cannabis with his local hospital or clinic. That's not a good career move," shares a Colorado physician.

The loss of federal funding is substantial. In the U.S., Medicaid and Medicare alone represented more than $3 trillion in consumer health spending in 2014. This represents 17.5% of the national GDP or $9,523 per person living in America (NHE.gov). For an individual hospital like Aurora Medical Center in Denver, Colorado that services hundreds of thousands of local patients, an annual budget of $220 million that is largely federally funded is not worth risking. The result is a lack of power and authority on the part of both physician and patient as it relates to this issue, as was expressed by participants in Chapter Four findings.

Medical Cannabis Evaluation Centers: A Fragmentation of Healthcare

States enjoying the financial gains from industry fees and sales tax from adult use decriminalization efforts (Colorado, Washington, Oregon) have pushed to "do away with medical cannabis [programs] in favor of the higher taxes associated with legalization," as attested to by all participants (12 of 12) residing in these states. Attempting to force "career limits" on the "number of recommendations a doctor can write during his or her *entire* career," is one action each of these states have unsuccessfully attempted, thus far.

> "If 100% of patients have an endocannabinoid system, then why should any doctor be limited on the number of recommendations he or she can write?"

When evaluation centers close and institutions prohibit recommendation support, patients are left without options. In Illinois, not having a medical cannabis evaluation clinic system has had detrimental effects on potential cannabis patients, as discussed in Chapter Four. As an example, in 2016 in Illinois, The eCS Therapy Center met with 1156 patients, who are interested in pursuing cannabis therapy but require a doctor's recommendation to proceed to registration. Of these potential medical cannabis patients, 982 (or 85%) are unable to obtain a recommendation through his or her personal doctors - or afford an evaluation center - given the state's policies (eCS Therapy, 2016 Mid-Year report). The majority desired the evaluation center approach, but found it difficult and expensive to obtain. The policies prohibiting physicians from recommending cannabis have largely contributed to the growth of this new healthcare sector. Integrative Cannabis practices are thriving, but under threat across the country.

Though hundreds of doctors may sign petitions in favor of medical cannabis initiatives, few are willing to buck the supporting healthcare systems and recommend it through formal channels once a program is implemented. For example, in Colorado in 2013 there were 19,897 actively licensed physicians (Young, et. al., 2014) but only 128 provided a recommendation to a patient that registered or renewed with the state's medical cannabis program during that year. This represents that far less than 1% of physicians are providing support to more than 115,000 patients, requiring annual recommendation renewals (Colorado Department of Public Health). Sadly, this trend blankets medical cannabis states.

Even private medical professionals must contend with institutional policies, especially if they have local hospital privileges. As one Integrative Cannabis physician shares,

> *Just putting your head in the sand and saying, "We don't know" or "We can't help with that yet," that's unfortunate. We need to educate and not be old sticks in the mud but take a new approach. It's not true that cannabis can't function and shouldn't function in medicine. The needs of patients that have medical issues are way different than people who just walk into a recreational store. They may not be able to walk, they be someplace like a hospital, a nursing home, or homebound. Medical care is a much bigger part of their day-to-day life because of their health issues. Cannabis needs to be integrated into medicine more directly. There are plenty of doctors who are willing to pick up the slack; who want to learn more about this and want to help. The system should be making ways to get more doctors involved. This requires some planning and some acknowledgement that this is an important part of health care.*

While instituted in the LR, policies that restrict physicians from recommending medical cannabis have great effect on the structural violence experienced within UR and UL quadrants by physicians and patients. "The Board of Directors of the hospital have decided that they are not going to utilize it or recommend it. Based on that, they also don't educate about it as a medical alternative."

Employment Related Drug Testing

States, like Colorado and Illinois, have deemed it inappropriate for medical professionals, specifically, or licensed professionals, like physicians, nurses, police officers and firemen (or others) to register as cannabis patients. Doing so, somehow authorizes policymakers to suspend medical licenses, because a physician seeking medical cannabis is assessed by politicians as being *too disabled* to perform their licensed, professional functions. Additionally, medical professionals are subject to employment-related drug testing, for new jobs, new positions, random requests, workmen's compensation related injury, and sometimes other reasons, due to institutionalized zero tolerance drug policies. For these reasons, it was unexpected to have a full third of physician participants (4 of 12) share personal experiences using cannabis. In fact, in the U.S. it has become difficult to enter a menial, fast-food job without being required to pass a pre-employment drug test - much less a professional position. Both physicians and patients have found a medical cannabis recommendation typically does not excuse the individual from a failed exam, like a prescription for Marinol (synthetic THC) will. Drug testing, specifically as it relates to employment or rather lost employment opportunities by patients, was a topic included in many participants' stories (23 of 32).

Loss of employment and loss of status with current or prospective employers (UL/UR/LL) were significant factors in participating patient decision-making (12 of 20). The extra-legal consequences of becoming a medical cannabis patient are real and are a direct result of the CSA and the division between federal and state policymakers. In 2010, Arizona was the first medicalized state to provide this type of protection to patients; however, few states have followed this example to include a protective provision in regulations regarding employment-related drug testing.

With the division between state and federal drug policies directly due to the CSA classification, federal contractors are required to drug test most, if not all, new employment hires for THC metabolites. Any individual testing positive to THC metabolites during a pre-employment drug test, for example, would be contacted by a physician representing the testing company. For an individual able to produce a valid Marinol prescription (again, 100% synthetic THC and Schedule III) will be given a *pass* outcome; for the individual registered as a medical cannabis patient, meaning a physician has recommended the use of medical cannabis (Schedule I plant) and a U.S. state has sanctioned this use, will be given a *fail* outcome, in most cases. Additional research into these issues would be valuable to future medical cannabis policy efforts.

Patient Rights

As discussed in Chapter Four, patient rights were mentioned by ten (10 of 12) doctors participating in this study. The two main areas of focus for physicians were 1) medical records and 2) drug testing by pain management clinics. Additionally, eighteen (18 of 20) patients mentioned patient rights in the two areas noted by physicians, as well as sharing, "healthcare and social providers not understanding I have rights as a medical marijuana patient." As both parties acknowledged during stories, patients often do not understand the rights they have to access or review personal own healthcare information or "are afraid to access it." The *Patient Rights and Responsibilities* information from Colorado's Aurora Medical Center (auroramed.com) are similar in nature to Patient Rights proffered by medical institutions across the country, particularly in regards to access to medical records and will be used as an example as they are very clear. Patients have a right to access and review personal medical records.

> *To have his/her medical records, including all computerized medical information, kept confidential and to access information within a reasonable time frame. The patient may decide who may receive copies of the records, except as required by law*

> *(Auroramed.com)*

Given that this policy is so transparent and universal, it seems odd to hear some patients feel "intimidated" by asking for personal medical records, but as one describes when sharing her story, it can cause UL fear.

> *The nurse was very insistent on knowing why - why do you need your medical records? Aren't they mine? Aren't I entitled to them?*

For some chronically and terminally ill patients this type of intimidation frightens them away from pursuing cannabis therapy further. "After all, if I can't get my records, then I can't get an evaluation center to recommend for me either. I'm stuck, right?"

In granting patient rights, the medical system also assures that collectively and individually, patients will:

    ✓ receive ethical, high-quality, safe and professional care without discrimination

    ✓ be free from all forms of abuse and harassment

    ✓ be treated with consideration, respect and recognition of their individuality

(Auroramed.com)

As well, they should "be informed of all appropriate alternative treatment procedures." Further, patients may "request or refuse treatment," although this right "must not be misconstrued to demand the provision of treatment or services deemed medically unnecessary or inappropriate." Based on institutional policies regarding medical cannabis recommendation, medical cannabis patients are viewed within these systems as demanding "unnecessary or inappropriate" treatment by engaging this "alternative therapy," as participants attest.

Medical vs. Recreational Cannabis Use

Policies in Colorado, Washington, and Oregon that decriminalize adult use of cannabis violate the federal CSA, like medical cannabis policies do. In 2015, physicians and patients, helped lawmakers understand, "maybe it is really medical. So, it survived as a medical system in Colorado." The medical cannabis program remains "under attack in Colorado" and has nearly been destroyed in Washington since adult use initiatives have been implemented (Jaywork, 2016). Oregon is now fighting this same battle (Vance, 2016) and other states will eventually follow, as adult use bills blanket the country during the 2016 election. An advocate and participating patient voices, "Every new medical bill seems to be entered into a big follow-the-leader game. Yet, no one is leading in policy, every state is failing miserably given the continued federal Schedule I status."

Though patients and physicians both find the disconnect between medical and adult use programs troubling, as shown in Chapter Four, both admit it "is helping attract patients that do not have cannabis experience." Since 1996, when California first medicalized the use of cannabis, the media began watching and sharing public interest stories, as well as news of D.E.A. interference, police raids on cultivators and caregivers, industry happenings, and any related crimes. Media attention has confused and frightened the public, from which registering patients and recommending physicians are part (LL). They've also had tremendous effect on public support.

Per the National Organization for the Reform of Marijuana Laws (NORML), 8 out of 10 Americans support the medical use of marijuana and nearly 3 of 4 support a fine-only (no criminal charges) for recreational users, according to Gallup and Pew polls (norml.org). Surprisingly, this support is growing quickly among pediatric advocacy groups as cannabis is a promising and probable treatment for children with epilepsy. In a 2014 Statement Summary, the Epilepsy Foundation states support for "the rights of patients and families living with seizures and epilepsy to access physician directed care, including medical marijuana." Further,

"The Epilepsy Foundation calls for an end to Drug Enforcement Administration (DEA) restrictions that limit clinical trials and research into medical marijuana for epilepsy."

Even the American Medical Association and other prominent medical associations issued similar statements over the years with little notice (Ingraham, 2016).

In 2013, *CNN*'s Dr. Sanjay Gupta apologized for his previous stance on cannabis that he shared in a 2009 article entitled, "Why I would Vote No on Pot." In an updated story, he publicly shares,

> *I apologize because I didn't look hard enough, until now. I*
> *didn't look far enough. I didn't review papers from smaller labs*

*in other countries doing some remarkable research, and I was
too dismissive of the loud chorus of legitimate patients whose
symptoms improved on cannabis. Instead I lumped them with
the high-visibility malingerers, just looking to get high. I
mistakenly believed the Drug Enforcement Agency listed
marijuana as a Schedule I substance because of sound scientific
proof. Surely, they must have good reasoning as to why
marijuana is in the category of the most dangerous drugs that
have no accepted medical use and high potential for abuse.
They didn't have the science to support that claim, and I now
know that when it comes to marijuana neither of those things
are true (Gupta, August 8, 2013).*

The first episode of his now series, *Weed*, had Gupta sharing the story of a 5-year-old girl, named Charlotte, a medical cannabis patient in Colorado with Dravet's syndrome and severe epileptic seizures.

Since that time, Colorado, as well as other medical cannabis states, has experienced an influx of *medical cannabis refugees*. The next section will discuss this phenomenon in greater detail; however, this broadcast and the change of heart by a well-recognized, public figure and physician has helped propel this topic into the mainstream, as has several reality television shows, like *Weediquette, Weed Wars*, or others, which publicize patient stories. A greater understanding about the experiences of physicians and patients engaged in medical cannabis recommendation conversations provides insights that will be helpful as public education (LR) about this issue emerges.

For citizens without experience using cannabis, the "media attention" and experiences they share of "friend and family" or other community members ("friends from church," "my son's soccer coach," "my aunt's neighbor") plays a significant role in LL acceptance or empowerment, and often is the trigger for personal research on medical cannabis therapies. Requesting a recommendation from a physician follows personal research. "You want to know it's going to be helpful before you ask your doctor about it. Why bring it up if you don't think it's going to be right for you?" However, as doctors and patients conveyed in Chapter Four, "Now that any adult over the age of 21 can try cannabis legally, many people who were too afraid to ask their doctor about it first, ask now, *after* they've tried it." As one Colorado patient mentions,

> "It is easier for some people to walk into a recreational dispensary with zero reference to what they will experience, than to sit down and ask their doctor if he thinks it will help. They know the doctor really doesn't know and let's face it, even I didn't want to risk that kind of stigma when I first came to this either, and I had some experience with it. It is frightening to get those words out of your mouth, 'Hey, doc, can you give me a recommendation for medical marijuana?' Real frightening."

A principal problem in states that have enacted adult use or decriminalization initiatives for both patients and physicians are the political attempts to "remove medical marijuana programs once legalization occurs." As discussed in Chapter Four, in 2015, after physicians and patients helped Colorado lawmakers understand, "maybe it is really medical" - it survived as a medical system in Colorado "barely." Washington has been less successful than Colorado, its medical cannabis program is hanging by a weak thread (Jaywork, 2016) and Oregon is now fighting this same battle (Vance, 2016), as noted earlier. Other states will follow as adult use (as well as medical cannabis) bills blanket the country during the 2016 election.

As a Colorado physician shares,

> *There was that perspective in certain quarters but I do believe*
> *that in 2015, through patient advocacy and other advocates*

*and at the legislative level, doctors spoke out - a lot of doctors
did get involved and spoke out in response to this perception.
Cannabis has a place in medicine.*

Finding cannabis' place in medicine has been elusive given that it still carries the Schedule I status, which assures it has "no medicinal value," per the CSA.

Medical Cannabis Refugees

State medical cannabis programs are emerging across the country. However, only 28 of 50 states and the District of Columbia have medical cannabis policies, meaning that access to cannabis for medical use is determined by your state of residency. As an example, residents, and therefore physicians, in Colorado have had access to a medical cannabis program since 2008. However, residents of Kansas, Utah, Wyoming and Nebraska, all bordering states, have no medical cannabis access. Further, U.S. citizens in Burlington, Colorado have access not only to medical cannabis with an approved state registration, but adults over 21 years of age have access to the decriminalized cannabis system since 2014. In contrast, citizens in Kanorado, Kansas, residing less than 25 miles away, face harsh penalties for possessing cannabis for any purpose. A misdemeanor charge, at the very least, can be expected for possessing any amount of cannabis. The penalties for simple possession could include up to six months in jail and a $1,000 fine. However, if the charging police officer believes there is sufficient cause to *assume* sale and distribution of cannabis might be an intent, the misdemeanor becomes a felony charge. In these cases, less than an ounce of cannabis - which is legal to possess 25 miles away - is now cause for up to 5 years in prison and $300,000 in fines.

Arizona and New Mexico also border Colorado, but residents of these states have access to medical cannabis programs; however, traveling patients commit federal crimes by crossing state borders and possessing cannabis in other states. Only six of the twenty-five (6 of 25) medical cannabis states, excluding D.C., recognize the medical cannabis patient status of registered patients from another state, but do not allow out-of-state patients to purchase cannabis within the state's borders (Arizona, Maine, New Hampshire, Michigan, Nevada, Rhode Island). As noted earlier, bringing "your own supply of cannabis means you broke federal law."

Further, Colorado's Amendment 20, as well as Amendment 64, provides counties and cities with the ability to "opt out" and not participate in the medical cannabis program. Though patients can apply through the state and doctors within "opt out" counties or cities can still sign recommendations, most don't because patients do not have local access to the products. "I have to drive nearly two hours to get to a dispensary; around here it's not like Denver, with a dispensary on nearly every corner, but that's what people think." Many Colorado medical cannabis patients are "inconvenienced" by local regulations, but believe those in other states are arguably more "disadvantaged because they have no access and it's still a crime - for doing just what I am doing ten miles inside this state's border. Twenty miles from here I am a criminal. It's just crazy."

For most patients, a desperate health situation has been the trigger for personal research. At some point, critical to the patient, personal research and desperation led them to relocate to another state for cannabis treatment. The term *medical cannabis refugee* was coined around 2013, shortly after the CNN "Weeds" show aired, "because that's when they began to arrive. There have been so many people move here just for cannabis, since that show, it's unreal." Thousands of families with children with seizure disorders, cancer, or other severe conditions and terminally or chronically ill adults have upended stable lives for a desperate chance to engage in cannabis therapy. 65% of patient participants (13 of 20) shared stories as medical cannabis refugees during interviews. As a participating medical cannabis refugee from Georgia conveys,

> *If patients had medical cannabis access in other states, they*
> *would not have to move here. If I would have had access in*
> *Georgia, I most definitely would not have moved to Colorado.*
> *My own state could have benefitted from my receiving*
> *cannabis and being part of the workforce again.*

Nine (9 of 12) physicians also chimed in on this topic, "since it has become so prevalent over the last few years." In a Colorado Integrative Cannabis physician's experience,

"Nearly every day I meet someone who has just moved here and is desperately ill."

The federal and state disconnect on drug policy is readily observable as medical cannabis refugees continue to flood in to Colorado and other U.S. states where patients can find refuge.

There is no statistical data that accurately identifies how many Americans are medical cannabis refugees. Media reports (*Fortune,* 2016; *CNN;* 2016) have noted that in Colorado alone, "hundreds of families have relocated from other countries." From around the U.S., it is many, many more thousands, perhaps, hundreds of thousands, in this researcher's observation (and as the founder of a cannabis nonprofit). This is an area of research rich for future exploration.

Rights granted to recognized medical cannabis patients vary considerably and do not extend beyond a state's borders, as discussed earlier. Because of the federal CSA restrictions on Schedule I drugs, crossing a state border with cannabis violates federal drug policy. As well, shipping cannabis outside of the state in which you reside is also a federal offence and federal postal violation. However, as this complex situation expands across the country, new problems emerge. A Colorado advocate and patient exclaims,

> I'm happy that there are doctors in other states that are open
> and willing to at least advise their patient on cannabis and say,
> "Go to a legal state. Go to Colorado or Washington or wherever
> you can to get the help that you need." I do get pissed off at
> states like Georgia that have essentially done medical
> decriminalization but are telling their patients - parents of
> disabled kids - to break state and federal law by going to other
> states to get the medicine and bring it back. Really, you are
> okay once they get back home but you are encouraging people
> to break the laws of my state?

As another Colorado advocate voices, "for resolution, the change requires federal intervention."

Black Market

Like the CSA, the black market is a LR system that functions all too well in the U.S. Though none of the participating physicians specifically commented on the black market when they shared stories with the researcher, beyond "patients tell me the black market is cheaper than dispensaries," nearly 100% of the patient participants (19 of 20) did voice opinions about it. Whether the home state had a medical cannabis program or both medical and adult use programs, patients share, "the black market is still thriving" in each. A recent Newsweek Special (February 14, 2016) suggests that in Oregon, "as much as 80% of the state's cannabis crops end up leaving Oregon. Much of this contraband is then shipped to the East Coast, where residents in states with high demand but harsh penalties, such as New York and Florida, are able to take advantage of the quality facilitated by legal cannabis systems in other states." However, while "it isn't difficult for some patients to find black market cannabis, for others it is nearly impossible." The one thing that's certain is that state-run adult use and medical cannabis programs are not game-ending competition for the black market (LR).

"The state-level policies and regulations are not competition for the black market." Yet, as more and more citizens move out of the black market and into medical cannabis or adult use markets "pressure to silence" and "assure invisibility" for dispensaries and ancillary businesses, like evaluation centers has become a focus of lawmakers.

> "Regulations like we have won't get rid of the black market. Decriminalization won't do that; only *real legalization* would do that and we're nowhere close to having real legalization."

As several Colorado patients share, "People still tell me they get their cannabis on the black market. It costs less and since our state doesn't require medical products be tested, though they do require recreational products be tested, who knows if what costs more is better for you? There has been some awfully bad medicine in these dispensaries." Though the black market remains an option, like another Colorado patient shares,

> *I had a lot of different experiences obtaining cannabis in the black market. It's an unsafe environment and I was wrongly self-medicating with cannabis in an unsafe way. I was self-medicating without knowing what I was getting.*

The divide between medical cannabis and adult cannabis users or recreational consumers is perhaps best defined as the difference between those who use cannabis in a focused, recurrent way (patients) and those who only use it casually for stress relief (recreational) (Nelson, 2015).

This section explores the federal CSA and its trickle down effects in the LR quadrant to State Public Health Institutions and local medical institution policy, including insurance company policies and practices that negatively impact participants. The cumulative effect marginalizes participants in medical cannabis programs across AQAL, as this section began exploring and the following sections will delve into further.

LL: Interior Collective

An integral evaluation of a metanarrative, where basic commonalities and relationships become more apparent among the multiplicity of perspectives or even customs of doctor-patient relationships (UR) provides insight into the culture of control (LL) storied by study participants in Chapter Four. Participants (32 of 32) relay, "We've been told that this is socially unacceptable." Though doctor-patient relationships occur within the UR quadrant, the LL and LR quadrants will have influence over the type of environment, atmosphere, and social space available, as well as the culture of the hosting organization the physician practices within. Kaplan (2005) calls these *invisible spaces*, as discussed in Chapter One. As participants conveyed stories, the social interaction within these spaces (LL) and the relational outcomes that result (UR) are noticeably influenced by LR policies and institutionalized practices.

Doctor-patient conversations about the recommendation of cannabis occur in these invisible spaces; between individuals who are products of cultural and social values and beliefs that may be quite diverse. Considering the doctor-patient relationship from this quadrant, along with the multiple perspectives of study participants, enhances understanding of the subtleties in play. Demonstrating LL awareness, a Colorado patient voices,

> *Something quite innate to cannabis that I've noticed with people throughout the world...cannabis seems to have an impact on us on the social level. It does seem to cause us to be more aware of those around us. As part of that process comes the sharing of our medicine, we share our life, what gives us life...that in and of itself, makes us more social. We interact more. We interact as we share our medication just sitting in a circle passing a joint brings us together socially. We interact and share ideas over that. There's something about when we experience a profound healing in our life, we want to share that with others.*

Common language, signs, and symbols that are understood and shared among humans characterize the LL quadrant, as mentioned in Chapter Two. To successfully rescript cultural beliefs about what it means to be a cannabis patient or to recommend cannabis as a medical therapy, a reflection on participant experience in this area is critical.

Goffman describes *normal* as incorporating standards from wider society and meeting others' expectations about *what we ought to be*. The concept of stigma is therein a device that ensures the reliability of the interaction order by punishing people who do not conform to current moral standards. Some cannabis patients note a considerable cultural shift in opinion toward cannabis users ("It's better than it used to be") while state policymakers push forward restrictive, prohibitionist policies trying desperately to satisfy growing public opinion that cannabis should at least be made available for medical use.

In contrast, others fear being exposed as cannabis patients with internalized (UL) and institutionalized (LL) stigmatization notably affecting quality of life.

> "I don't tell many people that I use cannabis. I don't want them to think differently of me."

Despite LR policies, LL acceptance within medical communities, professional communities, families, neighborhoods, cities, counties, etcetera, have yet to normalize the use of cannabis, even for medicinal purposes. While retaining vestiges of social disapproval that contribute to maintaining a "culture of control, the concept of stigma is therein a device that ensures the reliability of the interaction order by punishing people who do not conform to moral standards." Much of this stigmatization is conveyed and achieved through shared language.

Language is Culture

Language plays an important role in culture and cultural change. Words matter and can be harmful or empowering as demonstrated through participant narrative in Chapter Four. The culturally embedded ways of talking about cannabis as a Schedule I substance of abuse are stigmatizing and marginalizing for many registered cannabis patients and prevent most physicians from acknowledging it as a therapeutic agent or recommending it for patients. An insidious form of discrimination occurs when stigmatized individuals realize that a negative label has been applied to them and that other people are likely to view them as less trustworthy and intelligent, and more dangerous and incompetent because of it. "Pot doctor" and "pot head" would be examples of this type of labeling. As a reminder, Bottoroff, et. al. (2013) explore the patient perspective in the article entitled "Perceptions of cannabis as stigmatized medicine: a qualitative descriptive study" stating,

> *Even more problematic from a human rights perspective is the*
> *potential for discrimination in the healthcare system, where*
> *individuals fail to receive appropriate assessment and*
> *treatment for a health condition because of being labeled as*
> *drug dependent or a "pothead".*

The affected individual may act less confidently and more defensively with others, or may simply avoid a threatening contact altogether. The result may be strained and uncomfortable social interactions (UR/LL), constricted social networks (LL), a compromised quality of life, low self-esteem, depressive symptoms (UL), or unemployment and loss of status and income (UL/LL).

As one physician voices, "Some doctors just can't get over the things they've heard their whole career. They flat out refuse to listen to the evidence." This same language is deeply engrained in study participants, even those advocating for medical cannabis patient rights, as Chapter Four findings also demonstrate. Co-Intelligence author, Tom Atlee, states, "Healthy communities - perhaps even our collective survival - depend on our ability to organize our collective affairs more wisely, in tune with each other and nature (Atlee, p. 3)." This ability to organize our lives involves language. How cannabis, cannabis patients, and recommending physicians are represented culturally in language will either come to empower them or continue to marginalize them. The ability to understand life involves language and discriminating language can be internalized by the recipient causing a loss of self-esteem (UL), at the least.

Part of transforming cannabis care is finding new words to describe it's use. As voiced by patients: medicating vs. getting high; patients vs. stoners, are examples of how language is transitioning. How patients use cannabis can still be a taboo subject in communities or family groups. Educational programs for physicians and patients that include language components can "help demystify" cannabis use. "Doctors need to learn the different terms and terminology we use in the cannabis world. They can learn a lot of this by asking patients."

The type of stigmatizing language used to develop social constructs, like "stoner", is internalized (UL) and can be marginalizing and has extended to terms like "pot-doctor". As shown in Chapter Four, both patient and physician narratives contain traces of LL social myths and stereotypes. Another Illinois patient voices his LL experiences,

> *They are different with me now that I'm a cannabis patient. I had cancer and some days I was so tired I couldn't do anything; unless I smoked cannabis, in addition to eating it. My family kept asking me if I was just too stoned on those days. They've done that since I told them that I had become a patient and quit hiding my use. Before they knew I was using, for more than a year, they were commenting on how much more energy I had. Now I am just lazy or stoned, even though I am back to work since my cancer is in remission. It's just the way they are and the way it is around here.*

As demonstrated in Chapter Four, every participant's narrative (32 of 32) contains stigmatizing references. Several participants (17 of 32) share UL internalization. "It bothers me to be viewed as a stoner." Others voiced experiences of having negative labels applied to them by others: *Stoner, pothead, weed, pot* and *laziness* were the most referenced with 296 references in 32 stories. However, patient participants used the words: "marijuana, pot, or weed" within the twenty (20 of 20) narratives a total of only 64 times; the twelve (12 of 12) physicians used the same words much more often, for a total of 187 occasions. Demonstrating a change that is taking place, patients used the word "cannabis" a total of 214 times; physicians only 96. A Colorado patient says of her doctors, "It's just a daily fraternity party in their minds." To help others understand that,

"It is just plain prejudice; the belief that marijuana makes people lazy and stupid. Again, that goes back to a lack of education"

(LL/LR) and it is makes the medical cannabis recommendation process challenging for both parties, as this study demonstrates.

It is apparent that both parties are amid a language change. However, moving outside the cannabis community and away from those educated or experienced about the matter, most define cannabis via slang (marijuana or other terms) in order that they be understood. In short, the group doing the labeling separates "them" - the stigmatized group - from "us". In this sense, stigmatized people experience discrimination and loss of status. We reason that when people are labeled, set apart, and linked to undesirable characteristics, a rationale is constructed for devaluing, rejecting, and excluding them (Link, Phelan, p. 528). This type of language is stigmatizing in any community and can be internalized, as will be described further in the UL section.

Three of the participating physicians (3 of 12) had particularly stigmatizing language shadowing personal narratives, as shared through their stories. Interestingly, as noted in Chapter Four, all three of the physicians who are practicing within hospital or clinic systems did not demonstrate a transformative learning experience. An Illinois physician states,

> *They come to me and say they don't want to smoke it, but I think inside they are thinking 'Yay, I get to smoke pot!' That's what I think. Maybe not all of them, but a lot of them.*

Perhaps, these three physicians have not yet spent enough time speaking with patients using cannabis medicinally; each has been recommending cannabis less than a year. Future research that delves into the development of changed perspectives would further knowledge and understanding in this arena.

Another probable contributing factor is that each of these physicians is a Pain Management Specialist, meaning they work with patients that "often can't find any relief, no matter what we do." As one shares, "this means we deal with a lot of addiction." Though the nine other participating physicians (9 of 12) share a "belief that cannabis is a good for managing the withdrawal associated with opiates and narcotics," these physicians (3 of 12) have not established this belief. However, discourse like this "threatens the trust essential for a caring patient-provider relationship and may disrupt future care-seeking behaviour by patients as well as the delivery of efficacious treatments by healthcare providers" (Bottoroff, et. al., 2013, p. 8). How often it does is a question best left for more in depth research into the experiences of pain patients and physicians. The following section expands upon participant experiences with stigma related to illicit drug use.

Drug Use & Abuse: Myths that Stigmatize

As participants shared when they conveyed their stories to the researcher, social stigma regarding the use of illicit, Schedule I drugs are "one of the greatest obstacles" for either patients or physicians "to get over." Over the past three generations, the collective condemnation that "people like to get high" has taken on a negative, judgmental tone. The dominant narrative reinforces "the message that cannabis is bad." There are many toxic substances that people abuse in far larger numbers and with far more serious consequences than euphoria, like alcohol. Plus, plenty of pharmaceutical drugs also have euphoric side-effects; this is one of the main reasons they are abused so heavily in our society. The "Just say No!" perspective is deeply entrenched in American culture. As noted in Chapter Four, one of the private practice physicians espouses the dominant narrative as he shares his story,

> *It's just another way to escape. Some people use alcohol, some*
> *people use marijuana, some people use narcotics. It's just a*
> *mind-altering substance and people really like those.*

In the Canadian study discussed in Chapter One, (Ziemianski et. al., 2015), the greatest obstacle to medical cannabis recommendation was shown to be a physician's belief that patients are not actually seeking cannabis for medical purposes, but for recreational ones (p. 49), as shared above.

Other physicians (5 of 12) and patients (6 of 20) also have the shadow narrative of "people liking the escape from life and sometimes are abusing it because of that" embedded within personal testimony. Meaning 11 of 32 participants retain vestiges of prohibition - and related - myths and taboos within language. This internalized stigma

(UL) can be damaging in LL communities and UR relationships, like the doctor-patient relationship.

Myths about getting high are so prolific that they influence treatment. As mentioned earlier in Chapter Four, two of the physician participants (2 of 12) noted that they prescribe Suboxone to the medical cannabis patients that they've provided a recommendation to help them "handle the euphoria" and "avoid addiction." Suboxone is a CB1 receptor blocker, meaning it decreases the effectiveness of cannabis therapies by blocking the endogenous receptor system it stimulates, as well as reducing the euphoric side-effect. In other words, these doctors are prescribing an antagonist to the cannabinoid receptors cannabis is recommended to treat. This is counter-indicated treatment that demonstrates the lack of education doctors have received in this area. As a California patient shares,

> *My doctor told me I'd just get addicted to it. Then he gave me a script for Vicodin. How does that make sense?*

Sharing Dr. Amanda Reiman's work on cannabis as an "exit drug" (Reiman, 2007, 2008, 2009) through educational programs might go far in alleviating these issues, as will be discussed in the Education section. An examination of the Culture of Control participants experience will also help our understanding of educational and other needs.

Culture of Control

Participant narrative finds that due to LR policies, LL acceptance within medical communities, professional communities, families, neighborhoods, cities, counties, etcetera, has yet to normalize the use of cannabis, even for medicinal purposes. Stigma is typically a social process, experienced or anticipated, characterized by exclusion, rejection, blame or devaluation that results from experience, perception or reasonable anticipation of an adverse social judgement about a person or group. Per Wittgenstein (1953), "honourable upright behaviour, a staple of enduring sociability, is only possible if the breach of such norms is a realistic and publicly marked possibility."

Physicians and patients are both immersed in a culture of control (LL) as participants in healthcare systems (LR). Physicians, as experts, are viewed as *controllers* of therapies; patients, non-experts, are *receivers* of prescribed therapies. This is an ingrained cultural component of U.S. healthcare systems and it can adversely affect patients. One woman, a patient in her 50s describes the experiences that led her to cannabis therapy.

> *I did everything that my doctors told me to do. When I came to cannabis therapy I was on 18 different pharmaceuticals and was dying from the combination of them. Yet, my pain was so extreme, the doctors told me that I'd probably die within a year. That's what prompted me to find something better. I found cannabis. Now, I am off all those poisons, but for the remainder of my life I will have Lupus because of them. For the rest of my life I will use cannabis to help combat it.*

The request for a medical cannabis recommendation impacts the doctor-patient relationship directly in this space because neither party is certain that recommending cannabis is a culturally acceptable practice. However, for patient participants (20 of 20) it has been empowering to move from the *receiver* of therapies to either co-decision-making or in some cases, self-reliance.

Over two million U.S. citizens are medical cannabis patients, whose treatment relies little on accepted medical knowledge, but heavily on anecdotal information shared among communities of patients, social media, internet news, and even mainstream media. "When health practitioners are viewed as experts who tell you what to do, individuals become passive participants, blindly following protocols without taking authorship of their own lives" (Zucker, 2011, p. 133). Each of the participating patients (20 of 20) state "cannabis therapy has empowered me." An Arizona patient shares,

> *Something finally just clicked in my head: this is not going to work with the pharmaceuticals. You need to leave the pharmaceuticals alone. So, that's what I did. I found some kind of cannabis product to replace every single thing I was taking. I am not just using cannabis oil, I am taking edibles, I use dabs,*

> *I cook with raw bud, I do what it is that I need to do to handle the moment's issues, instead of going to a pill, I am going to the cannabis plant.*

Though this may seem like a random phenomenon to many, most patient participants (16 of 20) reported "getting off *all pharma*." 13 patient participants share, "Cannabis is my only medicine." But, even for those who have not been able to completely abandon pharmaceuticals, "a reduction" was reported by every patient participant (20 of 20). Recent studies support this outcome, reporting an overall 25% reduction of prescription pharmaceutical use in medical cannabis states (Lucas, 2012).

In the words of ten physician participants (10 of 12), collective ignorance and fear are the main components of LL trepidation within the medical community and an area education must focus on. "Ignorance and fear are to blame, which is probably true for all stigma." As a Nevada physician voices,

> *Ignorance stops conversations so that we cannot discuss and develop an understanding of what cannabis is and how it can be used therapeutically or otherwise.*

A Colorado physician shares,

> *If you just don't know, no one told you, no one told you how, or why, or in what way - how could any of this make sense? If you have never learned anything about it but just stick to social scripts of what potheads are and how they use it; you just don't know.*

As a society, we are having a hard time escaping old social constructs and forming new ones; ones in which all humans have an eCS and can benefit from *cannabis sativa* holistically, as can our earth and society.

The Cannabis in medicine: a national educational needs assessment among Canadian physicians (Ziemianski, D. et. al., 2015) elucidates,

> *Even more problematic from a human rights perspective is the*

potential for discrimination in the healthcare system, where individuals fail to receive appropriate assessment and treatment for a health condition because of being labeled as drug dependent or a pothead. In this context, patient-provider consultations become focused on extraneous issues, such as addiction and one's moral fiber, rather than the larger concerns of symptom management and the underlying pathology of illness. Amid this preoccupation resides an uneasiness and lingering doubt that CTP (cannabis for therapeutic purposes) use is contrived and manipulative, whereby cannabis is masking, and in many cases adding to, the individual's and societal problems. This discourse threatens the trust essential for a caring patient-provider relationship and may disrupt future care-seeking behaviour by patients as well as the delivery of efficacious treatments by health care providers (p. 8).

Terminally and chronically ill people often have difficulty sharing their voices. The results of this study provide an improved understanding of the many influential factors that are engaged within a recommendation for medical cannabis from both doctor and patient perspectives. That the outcome empowers *versus* stigmatizes patients often lies in the reaction of the doctor (UR). That the doctor finds education and empowerment within the culture (LL) and policies (LR) of the organization will in large part determine the exposed reaction to the request for a medical cannabis recommendation. "The patient is waiting anxiously to see how I will respond." As well, they are "visibly relieved to find that I will listen."

Loss of Status

Study participants (32 of 32) broached the topic of loss of status frequently within the stories each shared. The fear or the reality of derogatory treatment, like being fired from a medical practice or being labeled as a "marijuana addict" in medical records, or loss of employment as discussed in LR findings, were primary concerns. Both doctor and patient participants recognize that,

> "Obviously, doctors are afraid of giving a recommendation. They are afraid it will cause them to lose their license, their whole career, everything. You can't blame them for feeling that way."

This section will focus on patient participant experiences related to being "traumatized" or "fired" from a medical practice for requesting a medical cannabis recommendation or "admitting you went outside normal healthcare systems" to obtain one through an evaluation center. As well, it will expand upon the Patient Rights issues discussed earlier, as patient and physician participants discuss the labels of "chronic marijuana abuser" and addict. These were the issues most addressed by study participants.

Patients avoid losing status with personal physicians. "I didn't feel confident that my own physician would be willing to give me a recommendation…So, I didn't ask." Many participating patients (9 of 20) have been "fired" from his or her primary or specialty physician's practice, because they went outside the assigned health care system to obtain a medical cannabis recommendation or requested one from the personal physician. As one Colorado patient experienced earlier this year, when she "admitted to my primary care that I had my medical cannabis card for almost a year now. After he denied me and made such a fuss, I went to an evaluation center." She goes on to share,

> *I should never have told him! His not knowing meant I at least had some medical support. Now I have to hunt for a new doctor in my network. I am not sure if I should tell a new one that I am a medical cannabis patient. I don't need that to happen again.*

Experiences like this create distrust that affects future doctor-patient relationships (UR), as well the recipient, in this case the patient, may internalize the stigmatizing event (UL) or choose to conceal her medical cannabis patient status from future physicians (UL/UR). As demonstrated in Chapter Four narrative, the issue of medical cannabis is one of diversity that must be culturally addressed.

Other participating patients (7 of 20), as noted in Chapter Four, have come to find that the label of "chronic marijuana abuser" or "marijuana addict" has become a part of the patient's medical records. "I was very hesitant to have that on my medical records, which actually proved to be a wise approach." Participating physicians (5 of 12) also voiced concern about the "inappropriate labeling" of a patient, as well. The testimonies substantiate that these concerns are valid. As an Oregon physician shares, "marijuana abuser appears in patient records pretty frequently - placed there by uneducated and uncaring physicians, as approved by the administration. It really is horrifying." It is also highly stigmatizing and can result in the loss of status. In some cases, it also results in harsh consequences like the denial of life insurance, as mentioned in "Additional Findings" from the LR quadrant.

Medical cannabis use has also been responsible for lost employment opportunities, as one Nevada patient shares,

> *I applied for a job and a medical background check was required. My physical disabilities didn't prevent me from getting the job, but seeing "marijuana addict" from my primary care sure did.*

As shown in Chapter Four findings, the patient participants who are federal contractors (3 of 20) or veterans (3 of 20) shared UL internalized fears about this type of scenario (4 of 20) or had already experienced it (2 of 20). In the "Education" section below, this issue will be discussed further.

Importantly, when they first provided a medical cannabis recommendation, each of the physician participants (12 of 12) recognized that they would be learning from his or her own patients. In many ways, they express that they are "humbled by the opportunity to learn about this from so many vantage points." However, loss of status and discriminatory experiences have been a part of recommendation process for them. Collectively (LL) and individually (UL) physicians practicing in this area have been coined "pot doctors." This is a means of discrediting Integrative Cannabis practices and the physicians who operate them. Particularly within the local medical communities (LL), among peers (UR), and within medical corporations (LR), "pioneering practitioners take a lot of pot shots. Pun intended." Until the Schedule I status changes, "Not all doctors are open to listening about this." Those that fire patients from medical practices, certainly will not hear the voices, until "the establishment accepts this culture (LR)" and becomes willing to listen. As a Colorado physician explains, "Reefer madness is deeply indoctrinated into the medical community, there is a huge stigma associated with disrupting that."

Who's the Expert in the Doctor-Patient Relationship?

Doctors are experts in medical practice and medical professional culture but medical cannabis patients have become the experts in cannabis therapy. This is a disorienting dilemma because it affects the professional culture within the medical community (LL), as much as individual doctor perceptions (UL). More than two million U.S. citizens are currently registered as medical cannabis patients nationally and receive some medical benefit from that experience. Yet, few if any are considered experts on the subject. The anecdotal evidence they hold is overlooked and discounted as irrelevant because it has not been studied in the academy. Participating patients, like physicians are "frustrated that what we know isn't being tapped." As a physician voices, "Until the Schedule changes these patients shouting the medical benefits of cannabis will not be heard by the establishment;" therefore, they also will not be widely heard within the medical community.

What patient participants seem to asking for is an opportunity for *co-decision making* in healthcare decisions. A right provided to patients rather consistently in U.S. medical organizations through Patient Rights policies, but one that is seldom exercised. Co-decision making is an UR action that is dependent on the LL cultural support, and in this case, LR policies and regulations. Physicians and patients must both be empowered to share in healthcare decisions by the medical systems (LR), as well, this must be an acceptable practice within the medical community (LL). Circumscribing a treatment to an unwilling patient may have significantly less successful results than the physician desires. "I told my doctor I wasn't going to take those, but she gave me a prescription for them anyway." Patient autonomy and the subject of co-decision-making has gained a prominent position in medical ethics. It is generally recognized and implemented in health policies and contemporary clinical guidelines, like those adopted by Aurora Medical Center. The principles of patient-centeredness encourage patient involvement through shared decision making (Barry and Edgman-Levitan, 2012, Kristvik, 2011).

Unequivocal reports from observational studies indicate that a doctor-centered approach is tenacious and that patients still have a limited degree of participation in decision making (Braddock et. al., 1999; Campion et. al., 2002). Studies also indicate that preferences for being informed and participating in decision making vary amongst patients (de Haes, 2006, Swenson et. al., 2004). Elwyn et. al. (2012, p. 1363) explain,

"Some patients initially decline any decisional responsibility role, and are wary about participating."

Thus, the assumption within patient-centered approaches - that patients *want to* (and should) be involved, participating actively in decision making - has been contested in various ways. Additional research that explores co-decision-making in medical cannabis contexts is warranted.

On the other side of this situation, patients state they become empowered (20 of 20) using cannabis therapy. Some participants described it as "life-changing" and "my medical care was better because I became involved in it." As a Colorado patient shares,

When I became involved in my healthcare, it felt so empowering to wean the pharma. And, though learning how to use cannabis and how much of it to use was an experiment on myself, the better I felt, the more I researched and learned, and

183

the more I became involved in my own life. Cannabis therapy helped me learn to help myself. Now, I just don't accept and take the treatments my doctor recommends - at least not without a good discussion. I am no longer passive, I am involved.

13 participants were proud to share that "Cannabis is my only medicine." Recent studies support this outcome, reporting a 25% reduction in prescription pharmaceuticals in medical cannabis states (Lucas, 2012). 12 participating patients used the same inspiring words, "My body, my choice" to signify the empowerment they experience. For patient participants (20 of 20) it was empowering to move from the *receiver* of therapies to co-decision-making and "increased self-reliance."

Holistic vs. Western Ideologies

It is important to consider the cultural differences between holistic healthcare and conventional western or U.S. healthcare, as ingrained cultural ideologies have effect in the LL quadrant. The practices and premises of holistic healthcare differ from the conventional, Western medicine, insurance-driven healthcare market that physicians and patients navigate within the U.S. Defined by The Academy of Integrative Health and Medicine, "Holistic medicine is the art and science of healing that addresses care of the whole person - body, mind, and spirit. The practice of holistic medicine integrates conventional and complementary therapies to promote optimal health and to prevent and treat disease by mitigating causes." In contrast with conventional medicine,

"The most distinguishing characteristic of Holistic Medicine is that it is based on the fundamental beliefs that unconditional love is life's most powerful healer and the perceived loss of love is our greatest health risk."

Most participating physicians (8 of 12) repeatedly remarked that his or her approach was "holistic in comparison" with LR medical institutions and "normal healthcare communities." The other participating physicians (4 of 12) affirm a "holistic mindset differs" from the norm. In the U.S., traditional healthcare communities are heavily laden in allopathic culture. Allopathy is resistant to Holistic Medicine, which philosophizes that the "cause and cure of all disease lie within the body" (O'Shea, 2001). In contrast, the Allopathic culture has been taught to view disease as coming from outside the body (i.e. germs, virus, injury, etc.). The allopathic philosophy assumes that when "the body has symptoms like pain, fever and nausea, that means the person has caught some bug, some disease and needs to have these symptoms 'treated' - i.e. covered up. Usually with pharmaceutical drugs. If the disease localizes itself in one certain part of the body and won't go away, then that part of the body may have to be cut out with surgery" (O'Shea, 2001). Cannabis therapies assist with healing through inner body responses, which aligns well with holistic approaches, but noticeably clash with allopathy.

Patient participants (16 of 20), as well, comment that they are seeking "holistic care," in large part, because allopathy or "conventional medicine has failed." One Integrative Cannabis physician notes, "I have been working with predominantly medical marijuana patients for several years. Over 90% of them have chronic pain. I realized a few years ago that I'm basically doing a residency training program and a brand-new subspecialty of a holistic medicine." The primary objective of holistic medicine is optimal health and it is achieved through AQAL approaches and methodologies. As a participating Holistic physician and M.D. voices,

> *The basis of holistic medicine is healing. It isn't just about using*
> *herbs and acupuncture instead of drugs and surgery. It's really*
> *a focus on the different therapies and modalities - the diet,*
> *herbal medicine, acupuncture, and homeopathy; all of these*
> *things are great, we use them all in holistic medicine but that's*

*not the focus. The focus is on the whole person and optimal
health .*

A Colorado patient conveys,

> *If the medical community would focus as much on prevention
> and wellness as they do pharmaceutical treatment, we'd be
> closer to a holistic approach.*

Maybe this patient best sums up the collective consensus, "They have to want it - it has
to be a conscious decision in the doctor world." Collectively (LL) and individually (UL)
physicians must become less resistant to cannabis therapy, open to learning about
cannabis and comfortable interacting with cannabis patients. Support must extend
beyond individual doctors to the greater medical community.

Knowledge and experience with cannabis patients could change this collective healthcare
mindset. The patient-naturopath provided an interesting insight,

> *I tried to be a patient, but none of the medical doctors would
> certify me. That's back to that story of the resistance that
> medical doctors have to the stigma of cannabis. It took me two
> years to find a doctor...She and I had so much in common we
> decided to join forces. The situation with the medical doctors is
> that they admittedly don't know very much about
> cannabinoids. I was to educate the patient, prepare the patient
> for certification...and then the doctor that I was working with
> would certify them. This was a collaborative effort to give the
> patient advance support...I had no idea at that time that this
> would grow to be so well received by the medical patients...I
> have created a network in the community by educating the
> doctors to send the patients to me. Patients are referred to me
> for education, then I work with the doctor for ongoing
> care...The doctors like that I'm involved because I am the one
> who monitors the patient, watches their progress, and helps*

them with protocols or teaches other ways to manage their
condition or their pain or their P.T.S.D. The doctors are more
apt to work with me knowing that the patient is getting this
kind of support.

The researcher (as founder of The eCS Therapy Center) has also noticed that a social support model is well accepted in medical communities. But, without funding support, organizations such as this stand little chance of success.

Cultural Shift from Pharmacy to Dispensary

Resistance from the medical establishment (LR) and community (LL) can also be traced to the design of medical cannabis systems (LR). Nearly every participant (30 of 32) shared that "this new industry is way outside normal for medical professionals and patients who don't know much about cannabis therapy." The primary support proffered by the physician for cannabis therapy currently is the recommendation; rarely is it supplied along with education, consultation, or referral to a social service agency. These models still do not exist in mass. However, participating physicians (10 of 12) note that the dispensary model is also outside the norm for the medical community and "is hard for the medical community to accept." For several (3 of 10) this cultural shift "is hard to swallow." An Illinois physician shares,

To me it seems one step above drug dealer, the patient doesn't
have medical professionals to help them.

Another voices,

The dispensary model is okay for patients that have experience
with cannabis, but if you don't know strains, sativa from
indica, or how much cannabis is in an edible, then it can be a
not so good experience for the patient.

The testimony of participating patients (18 of 20) supports the physicians' comments about the collective failings of dispensaries. More than half of participating patients (11 of 18) find that "dispensaries don't have trained staff that can help you figure out what you need and how much you need to take of it." A common theme among patients is "I knew more than the associate [at the dispensary]." Future research that expands knowledge about how patients interact with medical cannabis dispensaries would be beneficial to system participants.

Lack of Social Support

Physicians and patients are both used to finding social support organizations (LR) and communities (LL), including support groups (LL) for patients suffering a great range of conditions. This is not the case within medical cannabis communities, because of the Schedule I status, there is no available federal funding and states have remained blind to these collective needs. A patient participant with a social work background shares the following,

> *Drug use should be a community mental health, not a law enforcement issue. We need to look at drugs as something that our society and humans have been using forever. In stigmatizing terms, being a cannabis user in this society is wrong...This leads to making people feel like they're not worthy or that it is a shameful thing that they are doing. They are not going to share it with their doctor when they can't share it with the people they love. It's still a shameful thing. We have got to take the shame out...Both HIV and cannabis use, they run the same gauntlet of shame. People feel that if they are using it they can't talk about it. People who are HIV positive also feel like they can't talk about it. They're going to be judged. They might be shunned. It is the same thing. People that tell their doctor that they use this and are told, 'I'm not going to prescribe your other medicine anymore' That is shaming! It takes away their option. Fear and shame become the reason they do not use cannabis.*

Many of the patient participants voiced experiences of shame that had significant UL effect. However, "several generations have been taught these myths" and have, in fact, helped develop the social constructs and stigma that surround cannabis use. "These are stigmas that have been put on this for a handful of years but have whole generations of our country thinking in one direction instead of understanding the smoke-screened fact that this is medicine," as one physician notes. Educational programs that demythologize cannabis use and which share current scientific facts and information, as well as patient testimony could help progress development in this LL quadrant relieving suffering for patients and physicians.

Participating patients (18 of 20) also found community in the "honeycomb of social media" (Kietzmann, et. al., 2016), as described in Chapter Four. Patient expertise is self-learned through a combination of internet searches, conversations with other patients, and embodied knowledge. All twenty (20 of 20) patient participants discussed in-depth online research that they had conducted prior to seeking a recommendation for medical cannabis, including the PubMed information shared earlier. Learning about the eCS and "the many ways I could use cannabis" was instrumental in his or her decision to seek a recommendation for medical cannabis. However, the support of social media communities could not replace family and community support, as the following section discusses.

Family/Community Acceptance

Social stereotypes about cannabis users, combined with continued UR and LL resistance within the medical community, and the extra-legal interference (LR) that many participating patients experience are all factors that have LL effect. For this reason, family acceptance is often a challenge for medical cannabis patients. As several physicians (5 of 12) note,

"Many patients have come to me and told me that they use it [cannabis] secretly because other family members don't approve or think they are going to get into trouble."

Time after time, "Patients worry about talking to their family or a religious organization, until they find out how it helps. Once they've experienced it they become much more open about discussing it with these entities." Embodied knowledge empowers the patients helping them reveal the medical cannabis patient status to loved ones. Though not every participant voiced having the support they hoped for, many were "surprised by the support of my family and friends." For others, the physical relief compels them to share their experience with others. An Illinois patient reports,

> They've all been supportive of me. I've talked to my family. I've
> talked to my pastor. I've talked to other people...I don't care
> who you are, I will talk right up and tell you. 'Look at me! I
> don't eat a bunch of fucking pills anymore! My kidneys aren't
> dying! That's great news, isn't it?'

Because *cannabis sativa* has been illicit for nearly 80 years and remains a CSA Schedule I substance, generational issues within families often affect understanding and acceptance. As a physician shares, "The reefer madness mentality is very strong still, especially with older people." Several patients affirm, "It's been illicit my grandmother's entire life, how is she supposed to know the truth?" Without public education, it will be a "long and intensive" research process for her to learn.

Several of the patient participants (5 of 20) mentioned that in addition to having a doctor-patient relationship with them, the doctor was also "in charge of" the healthcare of other family members. Some (3 of 5) mentioned this as reason for withholding the cannabis patient status from the primary physician or a specialty physician. For each, it was a point worthy of discussion as it presents an ideal scenario between a "previously undecided" physician and a patient "focused on medical cannabis" alternatives. As an Arizona patient shares in Chapter Four the experience can be positive, but for other patients it was unpleasant as storied.

I told my doctor that I had registered as a cannabis patient and a few months later he asked my mother how she felt about me smoking pot...I hadn't told my mother yet.

Given the Schedule I status of cannabis, continuing myths, and misinformation about its use and effects, as well as the failure to educate medical professionals or the public about the science that supports its therapeutic benefits, these kinds of outcomes are (not surprisingly) reported *often* in the cannabis community.

Education

As every participant (32 of 32) shares, "Education is the main thing that will bring change. Without it we will just continue to flounder out here." As discussed earlier in this chapter, neither state compassionate care policies, nor the Public Health Departments, which operate them, have any mandate to educate physicians or the public. "Regulated like outside systems that operate within an established system that doesn't want them," medical cannabis programs must progress. As well, educational funding and social support must be mandated and funded, "They go hand-in-hand throughout the medical community, except here." In consensus, participants agree,

"Education is, at least, the responsibility of the Public Health Department."

In fact, study participants, both physicians and patients (32 of 32) commented on the importance of teaching communication skills that "open the doctor-patient relationship to improved discussions" about disorienting dilemmas like this. Institutional policies and practices (LR) and collective stigma (LL) that has embedded in the UL individual are observable in UR relationships.

The following educational opportunities were conveyed by participants:

1. eCS-related Education: Required C.M.E. (Continuing Medical Education)

mandated for all physicians. Repurposing models from national HIV/AIDS Awareness efforts, which mandated physician education and training would help address failings in this area.

2. Use of Cannabis Medicine. The scope of dosing medical cannabis is outside the parameters of this study; however, all thirty-two (32) participants acknowledge its need.

Note: The eCS Therapy Center, operated by the researcher, is currently the only known NPO providing services such as this to medical institutions, physicians, patients, and the public.

3. Medical Cannabis Registration Process. Educational programs that address the LR issues described earlier by participants would alleviate "stress" and improve communication with the public (potential patients), instead of discouraging them as reported.

4. Cannabis as an issue of Diversity. Educational efforts in this area should include language and communication skills for both parties. "Courses on talking to your doctor are as important as courses teaching doctors about this [the eCS]." Participants suggest utilizing patient and physician panels, which help share both party's perspectives.

Educational programs that demythologize cannabis use and which share current scientific facts and information, as well as patient testimony could help progress development in this LL quadrant relieving suffering for patients and physicians. Charon (2007) emphasizes that "sicknesses declare themselves over time, not in one visit to the consultant" (p. 7), as do treatment capabilities for those illnesses and injuries. Charon suggests what she calls "narrative medicine" as a remedy for the type of healthcare fragmentation study participants describe. Narrative medicine provides a bridge for divides prevalent in medical care today, like those between the giver and the receiver of care, between the medical diagnoses of what kind of illness has affected the patient and the patient's own experience of illness, etc. Medicine, per Charon, inevitably has a narrative component that seeks to tell a story about how the patient became ill, what kind of illness has affected the patient and what kind of restoration of health is possible – and how.

In essence, healthcare can be analyzed as a narrative with a plot that is revealed in a patient chart. In some sense, the medical record is a type of literary genre, although it differs from other types of literature in that its primary purpose is descriptive rather than reflective. As Charon describes it, "Diagnosis itself is the effort to impose a plot onto seemingly disconnected events or states of affairs (p. 14)." The main purpose of the medical record or chart is to shape a structure based on the results of clinical examinations, the doctor's observations and the patient's own account of his or her sufferings – a structure that makes the patient's condition comprehensible and thus treatable. A medical diagnosis is, in other words, an interpretive act and just as every good novel is open to many interpretations, but not all interpretations, the patient's condition may also be open to multiple interpretations. As this study demonstrates, so is the patient's treatment. Future research that considers educational needs and a narrative approach may be highly functional in this arena as expertise lies within the patient population.

UR: Exterior Individual

An integral approach maintains that understanding any social phenomenon requires at least two fundamental dimensions of existence be considered. The quadrants can and often are causally related, such that changes in one produce changes in the others (Astin and Astin, 2001, p. 72). The four dimensions are interconnected and irreducible. The following section explores the participant's input related to the UR or Exterior Individual quadrant. The LL quadrant has already demonstrated the LR influence, participant stories will describe the realities of the LR and LL quadrants on the UR, more specifically. Through these metanarrative excerpts it is easy to understand how the LR and LL collectively influence the doctor-patient relationship (UR).

As discussed in Chapter One, Denzin (1989) describes a *disorienting dilemma*, as an "interactional moment and experience which leaves marks on people's lives" (p.70), though the mark may occur in the UR, the pain is felt and marginalization develops in the UL. The social stigma felt (LL) by participants, particularly as it relates to loss of status, triggers fear in the Interior (UL) of a person, which is expressed in the Exterior

(UR) through behavior or actions. In this case, the social stigma associated with cannabis use may cause a patient to fear asking a personal physician for a recommendation or admit they went outside "normal" services to obtain one, as demonstrated earlier. As participating patients attest (12 of 20) there is "fear and shame attached to requesting a medical cannabis recommendation" or admitting you went to another doctor to receive one. A Colorado patient describes,

> *It took me three years to tell my primary care doctor of ten*
> *years that I went to an evaluation center after he denied me a*
> *recommendation. I was scared he'd drop me from his practice,*
> *I guess.*

Given how many participating patients (9 of 20) claim they've been "fired" from a doctor's practice for obtaining a medical cannabis recommendation outside of regular medical care, these fears aren't unjustified. Baker and Watson's (2016) recent study, "How Patients Perceive Their Doctors' Communication: Implications for Patient Willingness to Communicate" concludes that if health providers are aware of how patients interpret expressed behaviors, "it may be possible to alter those behaviors in a way that favors patient participation in the consultation" (p. 634). Communication failures in healthcare settings (LL) occur between doctors and patients (UR). They are especially troubling because as this study demonstrates, they can result in poor patient care or patient harm.

In the average primary care appointment, both doctor and patient are rooted in social myths and perspectives (LL) and stigmatizing behaviors (UR) associated with cannabis use. The patient must muster the courage to enter a discussion (UL) knowing that the physician may change the way they view them (UR/LL), as well as be unsupportive or uneducated about the subject matter. In obtaining a recommendation outside of the established primary doctor-patient relationship, like through a medical cannabis evaluation center, the patient's desire to avoid stigma within this relationship often takes precedence. In the Canadian study discussed in Chapter One, (Ziemianski et. al., 2015), the researchers found that patients are far more likely to initiate the discussion about medical cannabis than physicians, for this reason. A medical cannabis refugee from Georgia now residing in Colorado shares,

> *I was shocked when I came to Colorado. I thought I was going*
> *to be able to go to my doctors and talk to them about cannabis.*
> *I was stunned to realize that they all had the same mind-set at*
> *the doctors in the south.*

Unfortunately, most of the medical cannabis refugees (10 of 13) share this experience, as shared in Chapter Four narrative findings and above in LR findings.

The stories of patients "being fired" or angrily leaving a doctor's service permeated findings. Avoiding the experience or "fear of disapproval" is the greatest reason patients seek a medical cannabis evaluation service (17 of 20). "The avoidance of shame" associated with a fear of loss of status (LL) are marginalizing to patients who already are suffering from terminal or chronic illness (UL). However, the physician's recommendation is a cornerstone of compassionate care policies (LR) that allow a patient safe, legal access and a small modicum of rights associated with the possession and use of cannabis.

"Without a recommendation, there is no relief."

Participating physicians (11 of 12), particularly Integrative Cannabis physicians (8 of 8) recognize the "flaws in this system adversely affect my relationship and ability to support the patient." As well, ten (10 of 12) physicians noted the larger systemic issue in domestic healthcare, that they could not provide adequate time, attention, and resources to meet the "real needs of the patients we're seeing." An Arizona physician conveys,

> *The main void I see right now is that patients come in and we*
> *have very little time with them. We have what I would call a*
> *segregated element of the whole medical system. We see them,*
> *determine that they meet criteria, fill out the paperwork, and*
> *that's it they're gone. We don't have a chance to do educational*

activities. We don't have a chance to see them back after we put them on the medicine, because after we've made the recommendation, they don't come back to us to get the product. They don't come back for another year until they have to be recertified. We don't have any idea how they're doing until recertification.

A Colorado physician affirms,

It's difficult to follow-up in a medical system that makes patients go outside their insurance or normal healthcare system. Educational follow-up like we do with pharmaceuticals is another extra expense that most patients can't afford.

She adds,

If you're going to do counseling and education that takes time and money. The patients are going to have to pay for that and they're not inclined to do that. They're inclined to pay for product but they're not so inclined to pay for additional counseling.

Florida's new medical cannabis program has begun implementing policies that will affect system participants. In short, Florida plans to require that every registered medical cannabis patient's physician provide an updated recommendation form to the state health department every 45 days; otherwise, access to medical cannabis will be revoked. As reported by a study participant,

If I relocate back to Florida from here, I will have to go through Florida's registration process, which appears to be a ways out. As well, I will have to return to a doctor every 45 days for an evaluation of my medical cannabis needs. For me and my wife, this means we will each need to pay an evaluation center doctor $30 to $40 per month, every month, until we can help

> *get this stupid regulation changed. Here, I pay $75 per year for*
> *one visit. In neither place, will my regular doctors sign those*
> *forms, so we must decide if it's worth it to return. I mean, we*
> *don't even know how long it will take that market to produce*
> *the medicine we need anyway, so we'll wait a while...or we will*
> *stay here.*

Several patient participants (6 of 20) comment about finding a positive doctor-patient relationship that meets current patient needs,

> *When you find a cannabis physician who is really practicing*
> *this, they make all the difference in the world. It took me years*
> *to find mine, now I wish she was my only doctor....and that my*
> *insurance would help pay her bill.*

The Integrative Cannabis physicians (8 or 8) appear to provide the type of service that is desired by patients (20 of 20). As one shares,

> *If I can learn their history, I can talk to them about each of*
> *those areas and help them get improvement on multiple levels.*
> *Because cannabis' different aspects can act on so many*
> *different levels, in the body, in different systems, when you can*
> *engage all of them you can really move forward with a*
> *person's health, their recovery, or symptom improvement.*

As well, each Integrative Cannabis physician expressed a key component to co-decision-making within the doctor-patient relationship,

"I am going to work with them to get their best result."

Stigma is internalized in the UL quadrant, but enacted through individual behaviors (UR), like those associated with either concealment or revelation. Many patients still conceal cannabis use from primary and specialty physicians. In fact, patients share that they prefer using a medical cannabis doctor or evaluation center, simply because they know they can reveal their use "without fear of retribution." A Colorado patient describes her UR interactions with her medical cannabis doctor,

> *The medical cannabis doctor looked at my medical records and immediately began asking me about different treatments, 'Have you tried this or that?' He suggested things I hadn't thought of and that my primary never mentioned to me.*

She adds,

> *When I got my last recommendation, we had a great conversation about juicing cannabis. We also talked about using THC as an anti-inflammatory. How that might be a good avenue for me to explore with my fibro pain.*

She goes on to share,

> *It was an interesting and informative conversation. One of the things that he suggested to me was to continue talking with other patients...to learn everything I could.*

She includes an important statement that reflects the positive UR experience,

> *What I remember most from that conversation was his availability to me to answer more questions.*

There are physicians who want to work alongside patients in this way, like the participating physicians and patients describe in their stories, it is a desire for both parties. One physician expressly states,

"I want to be able to [practice] directly observed cannabis therapy...bringing cannabis into a clinical

frame, as part of the encounter. There are a lot of potential legal barriers and that makes the stigma more."

When researchers asked patients how they make health-related decisions among the top answers were access to information, assertiveness, sufficient time since diagnosis, education, good interactive relationships with nurses and physicians, [and] encouragement by nurses and physicians to participate in health-related decisions (Say, Thomason, & Murtagh, 2006), as noted in Chapter One. However, when it comes to cannabis therapy most of these factors aren't in play. Biases, however, often are. As this patient shares,

> *If doctors could just answer questions based on the facts, not their feelings towards it, that would help patients a lot. A patient shouldn't feel like they don't have another route to take.*

For those who specialize in this field it is apparent that,

"There are plenty of doctors who are willing to pick up the slack and who want to learn a bit more about this. The system *should be* making ways to get them involved in their own practices and communities."

Most of the physician participants (8 of 12) had in fact, expanded a private medical practice "to accommodate those types of patients and help them deal with the rest of the medical community, who are very anti-marijuana." The others (4 of 12) are the rare in-house physician at a traditional medical institute who are allowed to recommend cannabis for requesting patients. Few individual doctors have stepped outside traditional U.S. medical institutions to specialize or practice specifically in cannabis therapy. A participating doctor shares,

> *The risk you take to do this, from being ostracized to the financial risk, is too enormous for most of us to overcome. I'm glad I did it, but some of my former colleagues think I have lost my mind and will lose my career. Some even think I've shamed the profession by helping these patients. I bet it all that they're wrong. I bet it all.*

Understanding the professional culture and stigmatization that accompanies these transitions will help others recognize the importance of this issue.

Co-Decision-Making

What patient participants (20 of 20) are asking for is support and co-decision-making with his or her primary and specialty physicians, as it regards medical cannabis recommendation, "not the cold shoulder." Physician participants (8 of 8) agree, "It's a model that involves co-decision-making and empowerment" that both parties are seeking. As a Colorado physician shares,

> *It's not like cannabis doesn't sit well with other health prevention: recreation, relaxation, stress relief and spirituality. Cannabis has many sides to it.*

She adds,

> *Even if a physician is not allowed to recommend it, surely he can ask questions and follow the patient's progress. When I started learning how patients were responding my beliefs were called into question, for sure.*

This communication requires an understanding of the AQAL consequences and risks and the type of skills that facilitate open conversation about disorienting dilemmas. Viewing cannabis as an issue of diversity, conveying knowledge about its use, and teaching appropriate communication skills to system participants would go far in helping resolve issues that plague medical cannabis recommendation.

Patient participants (20 of 20) desire a positive UR relationship with physicians.

"I want to have a relationship with a doctor that I can see regularly. I want a doctor to follow me and provide support."

As another Colorado patient conveys,

> *My knowledge on cannabis is extensive, but I'd like a doctor*
> *that will talk to me that is at least halfway educated so we can*
> *discuss details.*

For many patients engaging in the recommendation process is "difficult but if you stick with it, it does become empowering." A medical cannabis refugee living in Colorado explains,

> *I used to be the type of person who was quiet and took doctors*
> *at their word. I just figured that's the way it was. At the time, I*
> *was on 35 pills a day. I explained to my doctors that once you*
> *eliminate every other medicine, then you can't really contribute*
> *this to anything but the cannabis. Cannabis has helped me*
> *open myself and now I am working closely with my doctors.*

Both parties (32 of 32) do admit, "things are improving" between doctors and patients despite the LR and LL influences that impact the doctor-patient relationship in the UR quadrant. However, "education," like that discussed in the LL quadrant findings, "would be a great benefit for us all" and improve doctor-patient relations.

UL: Interior Individual

The Upper-Left (UL) quadrant references the interior reality lived by a person, as discussed in Chapter Two. Schwartz (2013) describes the UL quadrant as "posited as the locus of the master or key hermeneutic arena of perspectives; or, in greater balance, the lens through which the other quadrants are seen, interpreted, and evaluated" (p. 169). This quadrant encompasses a person's subjective personal experience. Internalized guilt, fear, or stigma has effect on well-being and personal decision-making in this quadrant.

For a chronically or terminally ill patient, it is an act of leadership to stand against social conventions challenging healthcare providers with a new proposal or your own embodied knowledge; an experience sought in desperation after conventional therapies have failed to provide relief. Further, it is an act of leadership for physicians to educate and act in ways that support the use of cannabis as a public health issue, while still faced with the reality that social policies and institutional policies concerning the medical use of cannabis inadequately address program participant concerns. The request for, or proffering of, a medical cannabis recommendation is a life-changing experience as described by the thirty-two study participants.

Internalized Language

Language plays an important role in culture and cultural change, as discussed earlier in this chapter in LL findings. Words matter and can be harmful or empowering as demonstrated through participant narrative in Chapter Four. The culturally embedded ways of talking about cannabis as a Schedule I substance of abuse are stigmatizing and marginalizing for many registered cannabis patients and prevent some physicians from acknowledging it as a therapeutic agent or recommending it for patients. An insidious form of discrimination occurs when stigmatized individuals realize that a negative label has been applied to them and that other people are likely to view them as less trustworthy and intelligent, and more dangerous or incompetent because of it. These effects from stigmatization are UL realities for the experiencers. Though many of the experiences shared in participant stories are shocking and potentially traumatizing, in many instances, "not everyone who is treated inappropriately is damaged for life, some rise up and move on."

A medical cannabis recommendation experience (UR) prompts people to think about personal views, beliefs, or traits and to consider what the views and beliefs of others might be. "It helped me do a lot of soul searching." Patients ask, "Am I a pothead?" and physicians wonder, "Do people view me as a pot doctor?" For those with weak self-esteem, an experience like the participants in this study share may be marginalizing. However, having a strong sense of self-esteem does not exempt you from an unpleasant experience (or disagreements, at the least). Over the course of time, participants "prepared for exposure" knowing the outcome "could go bad. But, I was prepared."

Bolstering this confidence was "a significant amount of personal research and a few trial conversations to test the water."

Skills and information well suited for public and professional education as recommended earlier.

Patient participants (12 of 20) share that being "re-labeled a patient vs a pot head" was part of the UL journey. As one explains,

> Being an undercover pot smoker for several years was like
> having two personalities - being a criminal and your family
> and friends don't know that it's you robbing the bank every
> night. [laughs] Taking a quarter at a time, no big crime, but
> crime. When I got that recommendation in my hand, I realized,
> I wasn't that. I wasn't ever that, but I was. I was buying
> marijuana on the black market from drug dealers. When the
> criminal label was removed, it was a huge relief. It allowed me
> to start talking about it. I guess now I've confessed my old

crimes to nearly everyone. Using cannabis - those were my
only crimes, I swear! But, they made me feel bad about myself.

Of course, the patient is still a federal criminal, in that he complies with state regulations, but not federal ones. The CSA (LR) bleeds across into UL experiences and leaves behind it's mark.

One of the Colorado physicians explained in Chapter Four, "for so many people the stigma is very large." The labels of lazy, stupid, and others are LL social constructs about cannabis users, except that of "criminal," which is LR, policy-driven and a living reality for many. For nearly 80 years, cannabis has been an illicit substance and in much of the U.S. this remains true. Thus, engaging in cannabis use is criminal activity, as is possessing or cultivating it in one state, but sometimes not another. As this study's findings demonstrate there is still a great deal of legal confusion in Colorado, Washington, and Oregon regarding the decriminalization of cannabis because of the conflict of the state policies with the federal CSA. However, if even seemingly, "Once it is no longer a crime, people are more willing to consider it a viable option." In fact, patients (19 of 20) confide they used cannabis prior to becoming a patient, stating that identifying "as a medical cannabis user was freeing." In some ways, it was "legitimizing of my prior criminal behavior. Marijuana-related crimes, access for myself, that's the only laws I ever broke and I did it on a regular basis for years, so learning and identifying my use as medical and getting actual relief was life affirming for me."

Stigma is a complex phenomenon expressed both subtly and overtly. It may be subjectively experienced in a great multitude of ways based on the nature of the stigmatizing condition and circumstances that affect an individual or collective group. Stigmatized individuals lose social status (Cumming and Cumming, 1965), they are discounted and discredited in LL contexts. They are seen as less than whole or are acceptable as individuals whose identifies are tainted in some way (Goffman, 1963). The reactions of others, as well as internalized self-feelings may lessen a persons' life chances or opportunities, including access to medical care. Stigmatizing experiences can lead to social rejection and social isolation (Goffman, 1963, Link, et. al. 1989).

One's perception of oneself is developed within AQAL [frames]. The LR, LL, and UR experiences of an individual and the context to the UL cultivate a sense of self. This sense of self can be rather pliable, as it is affected by all of life's experiences. The social epidemiologist Sherman James (2015) suggests that such fear sometimes generates harmful health outcomes. The extent to which a stigmatized person is denied the good things in life and suffers more of the bad things has been posited as a source of chronic stress, with consequent negative effects on mental and physical health (James, 2015). Stress is also associated with the constant threat of being stigmatized. Given that medical cannabis patients are already diagnosed as chronically or terminally ill, these effects can be deadly.

"I've already known four patients that died before they got a recommendation. How can anyone deny a Stage IV cancer patient a chance for relief?"

Physicians experience a great deal of career-related duress and say, "taking on cannabis was like taking on the world. It's stressful, but it's rewarding." As discussed earlier, educational programs for physicians and patients that include language components would help remedy these problems.

Isolation

Chronically and terminally ill people often become isolated, as shown in Chapter Four. A Colorado patient shares his experience, "As a patient, when you don't feel well you can't get things done. You stay home. Days turn into weeks, weeks into months, months into years." In fact, nearly all the patient participants (18 of 20) shared that isolation "had a particularly negative effect on their quality-of-life," at some point during a personal health struggle. Seven patients (7 of 20) specifically shared that isolation helped them conceal cannabis use.

"When I started coming back to life, my friends and

family were shocked to learn cannabis had *unlocked my door to fellowship*, so to speak."

Another patient describes her journey from pharmaceuticals to medical cannabis,

> *I felt like crap when I was on opioids. I really did! I couldn't sleep at night. I was on sleeping medication. I was anxious all the time. Worried all the time about pain, so they had me on another pill for anxiety. They put me on antidepressants. My body was so toxic from all of the drugs that I was on. I was walking around in a fog and didn't even realize it. I couldn't go anywhere or do anything. Now, the fog has lifted!*

Participating patients (19 of 20) affirm that collectively similar experiences are common, A participating patient voices,

> *As I started to feel better I became more active. I also spent more time thinking about my cannabis use, both current and past. I came to see I needed to get much more focused on how I was using it so that I would continue to experience improvement. That's what I did, I got really focused and my health greatly improved. I got my life back!*

Primarily what patient participants (20 of 20) described as most significant to UL experiences was the embodied knowledge they gained when they experienced the polarity between "the negative effects of pharmaceutical and conventional medicine had upon me" and the "positive effects cannabis has on my symptoms and my quality-of-life." A California patient shares a similar experience,

> *It's the side-effects of the prescriptions. It's been the medication not having much of an impact on the illnesses I have...that lead me to cannabis therapy.*

A New Mexico patient conveys a similar story,

> *I was a zombie for years. I had no quality-of-life. The pharma took away my will to live. It took away my emotions and just made me empty inside...With cannabis, I feel like a renewed person.*

The perceptual contrast between pharmaceutical treatments and cannabis therapy were startling to patient and physician participants and requires further exploration.

Beyond improved health aspects, both parties contributed narratives about "the more" of cannabis medicine. Many of the related stories will be shared in the section regarding Transformative Learning. "How it helps expand consciousness and extends to all aspects of my life." An Arizona patient shares,

> *It helped me become much more aware of the way the environment acts on health. Much more aware of how we impact each other and our responsibility to each other as humans.*

Another Arizona patient conveys,

> *Cannabis allows you to open up other pathways in the brain, other choices or decisions, it relieves the constant, mundane. It allows you to drift into an area of your mind that helps you know how to be a human. It allows you to connect with your spirit. It helps you understand how to be free. It can be deeper than that, but this is what it does for me.*

Given that the following section regards Transformative Learning and participating patients (20 of 20) shared a transformative learning experience, "the consciousness expanding properties of cannabis" may be helpful to marginalized individuals. Further research in this area is warranted.

Transformative Learning

An objective of this study is to determine if participants engage in *transformative learning* experiences because of engaging in the medical cannabis recommendation process (i.e. requesting a recommendation or offering a recommendation for cannabis). Thirty-two (32) participants shared narratives. 20 share journeys from chronically or terminally ill patient to caregiver or advocate or medical cannabis leadership. 12 physicians share journeys as a participant in the medical cannabis recommendation process, who have shifted beliefs about the use of cannabis from substance of abuse to medicinal agent.

The challenge of capturing a retrospective snapshot of the participant's learning experience was attained by narrative inquiry. As this study demonstrates, narrative improves our understanding about this type of social phenomena. The greater challenge for the researcher was to separate out what relates to transformative learning in contrast to what is a product of normal development of an individual given this context.

For the reasons provided in Chapter Three, a transformative learning experience was considered valid if a participant:

1. reveals a transformed view of themselves;
2. demonstrates a commitment to help others understand their new perspective; and
3. validates an improvement in communication contributed to the transformation.

As Commons, et. al. (1996) point out, during crisis points and "liminal" experiences, epiphanies have been shown to be a key factor in state development (Erickson, 1963, Commons et. al., 1996). Are those requesting or offering a medical cannabis recommendation at a gateway to a transformative learning experience?

Of the 20 patient participants, every one demonstrated each of these indicators; however, only nine (9) physician participants (9 of 12) demonstrated all three indicators. Eight (8 of 9) were physicians currently practicing in an Integrative Cannabis practice, the other is in practice in a university medical center; however, this physician entered medical school after completing a Ph.D. in Medical Geography, focused on issues surrounding medical cannabis. In short, because of his own personal experience, his academic, as well as professional career have emerged because of his "relationship with the plant."

More study is needed in this area to determine if these findings are consequential. It is possible that with further questioning, all twelve (12 of 12) physicians may have demonstrated transformative learning. But, given the context of this study, those practicing within conventional institutions (3 of 4) did not demonstrate all three indicators within shared narratives. Primarily absent from the testimonies were a transformed view of self and a commitment to help others understand a new perspective.

Reveals a Transformed View of Themselves

Much as findings in the UL quadrant demonstrate cannabis patients share that they gain a "greater consciousness about myself and others." Physicians shared how they were changed by understanding cannabis medicine, learning from medical cannabis patients, and in a few cases, personal experience using medical cannabis. One Colorado physician shares his experience treating shingles with medical cannabis,

> *You can get just so much from listening to patients and their*
> *stories. I appreciated it but until I had this severe pain,*
> *debilitating pain, where you just are completely consumed with*
> *it...When I had it myself, I realized what a remarkable healing*
> *herb this is...I saw right away that I personally was*
> *experiencing the benefits of medical marijuana.*

Unfortunately, few doctors have this type of experience to share. If they comply with institutionalized zero tolerance drug policies or state compassionate care policies that bar them from using cannabis, they cannot have personal experience using cannabis.

Another Colorado physician shares a typical story,

> *I am someone who came to cannabis medicine, who had a very*

conventional background, a very solid research-based background, but I had become alternative minded through an evolution and understanding of medicine.

She goes on to share,

I am very curious. I think that's a piece of it; as far as me being able to be more engaged with the patients perhaps than some other doctors doing cannabis medicine...It's totally new for doctors to be practicing...to be able to personally hear from my patients, learn what they are noticing and observing, and to learn those clinical patterns has been an incredible opportunity...I didn't know it at first, but humanity is crying out for cannabis!

Commons et. al. (1996) point out that during crisis points and "liminal" experiences, epiphanies have been shown to be a key factor in state development (Erickson, 1963, Commons et. al., 1996), much as this physician describes experiencing.

Are those requesting or offering a medical cannabis recommendation at a gateway to a transformational learning experience? For patients (20 of 20), the UL awareness was "life-changing." Not only have they found some symptom-relief to aid in recovery, but "being given an opportunity to be someone besides a bed-ridden, chronically ill nobody, changed my life. I am still chronically ill but I am functioning and feeling better about myself." An Arizona patient shares,

This subject just makes me want to put my social justice boots on! Holding the results in people's faces and saying, 'This is what is happening. You need to be on-board with this! It needs to be a decision and a choice for people. It has to be available.

Demonstrates a Commitment to Help Others Understand Their New Perspective

Elizabeth Lange (2004) finds transformative learning "is not just an epistemological process involving a change in worldview and habits of thinking, it is also an ontological process where participants experience a change in their being in the world including their forms of relatedness" (p. 137). The relationship between transformation and action is supported by other scholars (Courtenay et. al., 2000; Baumgartner, 2002; Garvett, 2004) and was evident within participant narratives. As shared, patient participant actions demonstrate commitment to help others understand a newly developed perspective on cannabis. For example, an Illinois patient conveys, "If I can make it easier for anyone down the road, I am happy to do what I can to further their understanding." An Arizona patient also shares,

> I started volunteering my time, working with patients to help them get medication, to answer questions, to make the whole experience less stressful. So many people are grateful for a space they can come and be social with other people. Being with others calms the anxiety about it. When we're able to share our experiences with other people, it is a calming mechanism for us all.

For patient participants, particularly, activism in the medical cannabis arena is a result of a transformed view of themselves and "improved health that allows me to get out and share my voice."

Validates an Improvement in Communication Contributed to the Transformation

Paradigmatic shifts in communication are becoming more readily observed in the cannabis community among doctors and patients. As both parties (32 of 32) share, "Things are getting better out there." However, as Taylor elucidates, "The often-unquestioned celebratory nature of transformative learning and the overlooked negative consequences, both personally and socially, of a perspective transformation" must be considered as they relate to the issue of medical cannabis. Though transformative learning experiences are often linked to *leadership development*, a positive expression of the event, *marginalization* is also a probable negative outcome, much as this study's findings expose. However, this study also finds that despite apparent marginalization patients engaging in cannabis therapy experience transformative learning. In many cases, patients (20 of 20) are empowered by these adverse experiences and these experiences guided them toward a leadership position in the medical cannabis community.

Patients (20 of 20) also recognized that in gaining voice, "I realized that I could be a voice for a lot of different people." As an Illinois patient shares,

> "When the world catches hold of this they will be like me, they won't be able to let it go. Once I learned and overcame the fear, it was on!"

A Colorado patient decided to act on behalf of others,

> *The governor set up a task force with no patient representative on it. I went to the very first task force meeting. I ran the governor and the task force up one side and down the other for not having a patient representative. I told them then it was my job and that I was going to be there, at every meeting, to make sure that patients were represented...I am not up there for my own ego, for myself. My first priority has always been the patient and what patients need - making sure their voices are included.*

Understanding "myself and cannabis therapy more helped me develop the courage to share my voice for those too afraid to do so."

Physicians also share stories of patients "enthusiasm and activism" though few (3 of 9) spoke of personal activism in this arena. However, they admit "It is in the hearing and telling of these stories that change occurs," in one physician's words. In another's, "Patients are very compelled to tell others about their experience with this medicine." A Colorado physician shares,

> Some of these patients have such moving stories. They are sharing these stories with lawmakers and the public in ways that are changing things positively. Every chance I get I tell other medical professionals these stories. It's like planting discussion seeds.

Further, she adds,

> It's hard to argue with first-person testimony and sharing my patient's stories helps others understand why this has become so important to me. Though it seems out of character that I am working with marijuana, I am doing it because it helps my patients.

For most doctors and patients, the recommendation of cannabis is a paradigmatic shift that has AQAL effect.

Mezirow (1991, 2000) led the field of transformative learning research offering a theory of learning that is "uniquely adult, abstract and idealized, grounded in the nature of human communication" (Taylor, 1998, p. 173). The theory of transformative learning has been a focus of research in medical education, cooperative extensions, health education, educational administration, and communications; as a theory, it is relevant to this project. Transformative learning theory is developmental in nature, it explores learning as the "process of using a prior interpretation to construe a new or revised interpretation of the meaning of one's experience in order to guide future action" (Mezirow, 1996, p. 162).

During transformative learning experiences,

individuals reevaluate assumptions and gain "a more dependable frame of reference...one that is more inclusive, differentiating, permeable (open to other viewpoints), critically reflective of assumptions, emotionally capable of change, and integrative of experience"

(Mezirow, 2000, p. 19 in Baumgartner, 2002, p. 44). Paradigmatic shifts such as this are becoming more readily observed in the cannabis community among doctors and patients and require further exploration.

Future Research and Education

This study's findings have implications beyond gaining an understanding of the medical cannabis recommendation process as experienced by system participants. In particular, the use of integral theory and the AQAL frame can be useful in community-based trials that used mixed methods to reach clinical research goals and objectives. As discussed in Chapter One, EBM requires clinicians to define a clinical question, assemble the evidence, appraise the evidence, and apply the evidence while considering their experiences as a medical practitioner and their patients' individual circumstances ("Evidence based medicine: what it is and what it isn't," 1996). As an interdisciplinary researcher, I believe we can either preserve the status quo or look for new ways to help medical practitioners gain valid knowledge about cannabis as a therapeutic agent. Integral approaches provide a solid frame and help assemble, appraise, and apply the evidence while still considering the experiences of system participants, as this study demonstrates. Integral medicine requires integral approaches.

Findings also demonstrate that narrative inquiry can be powerful in the social sciences, public policy, leadership, and other disciplines. As shared, a great deal of data exists in patient testimony that validates Charon's long held premise that narrative could also be useful in clinical trials, specifically in community-based clinical efforts in this arena, as well as many others (Charon, 2001, p. 1900). Viewing cannabis as an issue of diversity, conveying knowledge about its use, and teaching appropriate communication skills to system participants would go far in helping resolve issues that plague medical cannabis recommendation, as this study's participants voice.

Over two million U.S. citizens are currently registered as medical cannabis patients and are now receiving some medical benefit from that experience. Yet, few if any are considered experts on the subject. The anecdotal evidence they hold is overlooked and discounted as irrelevant because it has not been studied in the academy. Yet, this study validates this knowledge is important and much can be learned from it. Participants share frustration that "what we know isn't being tapped." Participating in narrative inquiry empowers patients.

"It feels so good to finally share my story with someone."

Data related to patient cannabis use, specifically dosing cannabis products, was excluded from this study, as were the medical histories of patient participants. Though the data was rich, it was not relevant to the study-at-hand. However, the depth of data collected suggests that narrative inquiry could help fill the gaps in knowledge related to dosing medical cannabis, an issue of importance raised by both physician and patient participants. The eCS Therapy Center is among the first NPOs to offer patient, public, and medical professional education and training that addresses the topic of dosing and provides targeting dosing guidelines to medical cannabis patients.

Future interdisciplinary studies, using mixed methods, perhaps incorporating narrative inquiry from patient journal texts, as well surveys or other pertinent instruments that combine the clinical approaches desired by the medical establishment and the narratives of those experiencing the therapy and treatment process are possible utilizing a narrative approach. Narrative inquiry that seeks to expose how patients choose cannabis therapy and their experiences as medical cannabis patients can provide the academy with insights as to how and why this *new phenomenon* is gaining credibility and public attention.

Contrast between pharmaceutical treatments and cannabis therapy are another startling area in need of further exploration. Given that millions of Americans have embodied experience using cannabis therapeutically and studies report significant reduction of pharmaceutical use in medicalized states (Lynch and Clark, 2003), much can be learned from patients that can be shared via educational efforts with the medical establishment and public. Charon (2001) suggests,

"Programs have been under way for some time in incorporating narrative work into many aspects of medical education and practice. The teaching of literature in medical schools has become widely accepted as a primary means to teach about the patient's experience and the physician's interior development."

(p. 1900). Participant suggestions of instructional guides, "factual public service announcements," continuing medical education courses, and other "public health support that is given to normal health programs" would go a long way to remedying concerns brought by this study's participants and system participants at large. Along with such outcomes, "research are scholarly efforts to uncover the basic mechanisms, pathways, intermediaries, and consequences of narrative practices, supply the "basic science" of theoretical foundations and conceptual frameworks for these new undertakings (p. 1900). Educational funding must be mandated and made available for medical cannabis programs, so that system participants can be served appropriately. In consensus, study participants (32 of 32) shared that education, "which is often reliant on research, of course," is the greatest area of need.

This study also demonstrates research that explores co-decision-making in healthcare contexts is warranted. Co-decision making is an UR action that is dependent on the LL cultural support and LR policies and regulations. Physicians and patients must be empowered to share in healthcare decisions by the medical systems (LR), as well this must be an acceptable practice within the medical community (LL). Exploring co-decision making through medical cannabis contexts can improve healthcare systems for all participants.

In Chapter Four, one of the Colorado physicians shares that "for so many people the stigma is very large" and other study participants affirm this position. Particularly, the labels of lazy or stupid are LL social constructs about cannabis users that have strong UL effect among participants. Hathaway, et al (2012) share, "Terms like 'pothead', 'druggie', and other demeaning labels were deemed by the respondents to be based on misconceptions that betray a lack of knowledge of the drug and its effects" (p. 458). This study's participants affirm this position. Moving from assumptions that are commonly endorsed (i.e. amotivational or lazy) to newly identified or stereotypically rejected (i.e. productive or focused) is possible if we examine attitudes on deviance, dependence, and views about the fulfillment of expected social roles in relation to cannabis use in more depth, particularly related to the therapeutic experience of patients. Research projects which consider the social constructs versus the lived experience of cannabis patients can assist with the normalization of cannabis use. Combined with educational efforts, increasing the knowledge about cannabis as an issue of diversity would help change dominant public narratives.

The connection between cannabis and other illicit drug use is clearly still a source of stigma in the lives of study participants and can be easily observed in the dominant public discourse regarding medical cannabis. The sections "Medical Versus Recreational Cannabis Use" (LR) and "Drug Use & Abuse: Myths that Stigmatize" (LL) share participant concerns that support the need for additional inquiry. When considered along with Reiman's (2009) work on cannabis as an "exit drug" for opiate, narcotic, and alcohol addictions, it becomes obvious that this is another arena requiring additional research efforts. Narrative inquiry into the experiences of those recovering from illicit or other drug dependencies may be beneficial in learning more about the role of cannabis

217

in their substance abuse and recovery experiences. This type of inquiry may also explain and clarify how the use of cannabis differs from other illicit or Schedule I substances.

The presumption that the use of cannabis is incompatible with conventional responsibilities and roles (i.e. doctor, patient, parent) is another area in need of academic exploration. For instance, this study demonstrates, medical cannabis system participants are negatively impacted in employment-related roles and contexts. Future public policy efforts require that zero drug tolerance policies and other employment and healthcare related policies regarding Schedule I drugs to be reevaluated and assessed. Social systems from public schools to housing to most public support services comply with the CSA and their policies adversely impact medical cannabis patients, like Ashley Weber and Daisy Bram, as mentioned in Chapter One. Research must begin to explore within the plethora of disciplinary and interdisciplinary opportunities revealed by this social phenomenon.

Finally, the value of gaining even a small glimpse of the issue of transformative learning in relation to participants in medical cannabis systems, healthcare systems, communities, and other relationships encourages future research to determine whether this phenomenon is indeed prevalent within the cannabis community. Understanding how and why system participants engage in transformative learning may help educators develop successful programs that begin to fill the vast gap participants describe. This study chose not to use levels of develop assessment to determine participant levels of ego development. It would be interesting to consider transformative learning and ego development in relation to the development of leadership skill in future study. Also, exploration into "the consciousness expanding properties of cannabis" may be helpful to marginalized individuals, particularly how the terminally and chronically ill are affected by this side-effect.

The arena of medical cannabis is new to research study, particularly outside the hard sciences focused on learning about the endocannabinoid system. This study is among the earliest in the social sciences. For this reason, there is infinite potential for research should funding be made available through normal channels. Until that time, few academics tread into this arena because of the funding restrictions; it simply isn't worth the fight. In the six years of Ph.D. studies at Union Institute and University, I have been honored to be recognized in 16 peer-reviewed events, through publishing and presentation. However, funding for research projects, scholarships, and fellowships has been practically nonexistent, in large part due to my topic of interest. Though this situation seems to be changing institutional support for studies in this area may also be problematic for some time to come.

Conclusion

The physician's recommendation is a cornerstone of compassionate care policies that allow a patient safe, legal access and a small modicum of rights associated with the possession and medical use of cannabis. Patients should be able to discuss a medical cannabis recommendation with personal primary and specialty care physicians without fear of stigmatization or loss of status; as well, physicians should have information about the eCS and the use of cannabis to share with patients. This, however, is not the reality medical cannabis program participants experience currently. As this study explores, the U.S. Controlled Substances Act conflicts with state-level compassionate care policies causing system participants undue hardship and stigmatization. Understanding the experiences of system participants is critical to the academy, policymakers, medical cannabis program participants, and the public. This study is among the first to illuminate the experiences of system participants in these medical cannabis programs.

In understanding the life experience of an individual doctor or patient, the UL or internal, subjective meaning-making, and UR or objective actions and behaviors are relevant; as well the context of LR or objective systems and LL or collective cultural and meaning-making systems, are also influential. In this exploration, an integral understanding was developed from a narrative analysis on the subjective meaning to individual doctors and patients (UL); observations and demonstrations of individual behaviors shared narratively (UR); discussing tools and processes to be used on the collective level (LR), and the uncovering of social and cultural characteristics that affect the conversation about medical cannabis recommendation (LR/LL). This study supports, as well as helps readers understand the significance of the experiences system participants face. It provides a clearer understanding through conveyed experiences of

219

those requesting or offering a medical cannabis recommendation affect include the myriad of factors they consider before making this decision.

Medical practice, as well as the lives of patients and physicians, unfold in a series of complex narrative situations; including those between the doctor and patient, the physician and him or herself, the physician and colleagues, patient or physician with family, friends, and cultural groups or greater society. Understanding how medical cannabis is affecting society and beginning with doctor-patient relationships exposes us to many areas in need of attention. Stigma has been demonstrated to have a negative impact on social interaction (UR/LL), employment opportunities (LR/LL), emotional well-being (UL), and self-perceptions (UL) (Link, et. al. 1997).

The following themes were exposed early in the data collection process:

1) The federal CSA has trickledown effect in the LR quadrant to State Public Health Institutions and local medical institution policy. The cumulative effect marginalizes and affects decision-making for system participants across AQAL.

2) Society, and therefore, communities and cultures are transitioning to new social constructs about what it means to use cannabis (LL) and to be a cannabis user (UL). At this critical juncture, public and professional education and social support are necessary for participants in medical cannabis systems and communities.

3) The doctor-patient relationship is directly and negatively impacted by the CSA, and the LR debris it causes. A frequent and costly side-effect is fragmentation of patient care and disruption of doctor-patient relations (UR).

4) Cultural perceptions (LL) about alternative healthcare, Holistic Medicine, and substance abuse and addiction seep heavily into myths and taboos about cannabis use.

5) Physicians and patients have both experienced internalized fear, loss of status, stigmatizing judgment, and have been denied personal expression (UL) because of the continued prohibition of cannabis the CSA reinforces.

6) Transformative learning experiences are common within the medical cannabis community, as observed and exhibited in participant stories.

It is an act of leadership for physicians to act in ways that support the recommendation of medical cannabis, educate patients, and support this dilemma as a public health issue, while still faced with the reality that our social policies and sometimes institutional policies concerning the medical use of cannabis are inadequate. It is also an act of leadership for patients to educate others, including personal physicians, and act in ways that support cannabis as a public health issue, while facing individualized and collective stigma. Medicine, is an enterprise in which one human being (physician) extends help to another (patient). As such, it is always grounded in the subjective and intersubjective domains (UL, LL); as well, the intersubjective is always affected by the objective and interobjective (UR, LR), all of which is readily revealed through narrative.

Every study participant (32 of 32) emphatically voiced the need for public, patient, physician, and medical institutional education. Patients (20 of 20) and some physicians (9 of 12) also suggest medical cannabis education be extended to public policy leaders (i.e. congress, city council, county commission, police and social agencies were specifically noted) and others "in need of truth." The following educational opportunities were conveyed by participants and begin to address the educational void in the area of medical cannabis recommendations:

1) eCS-related Education: Required C.M.E. (Continuing Medical Education) mandated for all physicians. Repurposing models from national HIV/AIDS Awareness efforts, which mandated physician education and training would help address failings in this area.

2) Use of Cannabis Medicine. The scope of dosing medical cannabis is outside the parameters of this study; however, all thirty-two (32) participants acknowledge its need.

3) Medical Cannabis Registration Process. Educational programs that address the LR issues described earlier by participants would alleviate "stress" and improve communication with the public (potential patients), instead of discouraging them as reported.

4) Cannabis as an issue of Diversity. Educational efforts in this area should include

language and communication skills for both parties. "Courses on talking to your doctor are as important as courses teaching doctors about this." Participants suggest utilizing patient and physician panels, which help share both parties' perspectives.

Educational programs that demythologize cannabis use and which share current scientific facts and information, as well as patient testimony, could help progress development in this LL quadrant, thereby relieving suffering for patients and physicians.

References

(2016, February 14). Pot is still lighting up the black market. Newsweek Special Edition. Retrieved from: http://www.newsweek.com/weed-black-market-424706

(2016, August 11). Here's what the DEA said about marijuana today. *Fortune Online*. Retrieved from: http://fortune.com/2016/08/11/marijuana-restrictions-classification/

Aggarwal, S., et. al. (2009). Medicinal use of cannabis in the United States: Historical perspectives, current trends and future directions. *Journal of Opioid Management*. 5(3), 153-168.

Alexander, M. (2012). *The New Jim Crow: Mass incarceration in the age of colorblindness*. New York: The New Press.

Andriote, J.M. (1999). *Victory deferred: How AIDS changed gay life in America*. Chicago: University of Chicago Press.

Annas, G.J. (2014). Medical marijuana, physicians and state law. *The New England Journal of Medicine. 371*(11), 983-985.

Bachhuber, M.A., et. al. (2014) Medical cannabis laws and opioid analgesic overdose mortality in the United States, 1999-2010. *JAMA Internal Medicine. 174*(10), 1668-1673.

Baker, D., Pryce, G., Giovannoni, G., & Thompson, A.J. (2003). *The therapeutic potential of cannabis.* Washington, D.C.: U.S. Government Printing Office.

Baker, S. & Watson, B. (2015). How patients perceive their doctors' communication: Implications for patient willingness to communicate. *Journal of Language and Social Psychology. 34*(6), 621-639.

Barnes, B., Bloor, D., & Henry, J. (1996). *Scientific knowledge: A sociological analysis.* Chicago: University of Chicago Press.

Barnwell, S., Smuckers, B. Earleywine, M. & Wilcox, R. (2006). Cannabis, motivation, and life satisfaction in an internet sample. *Substance Abuse Treatment, Prevention, and Policy. 1*(1), 1.

Baumgartner, I, (2002). Living and learning with HIV/AIDS: Transformational tales continued. *Adult Education Quarterly. 54*, 44-70.

Beck, D., Dossey, B., & Rushton, C. (2011). Integral nursing and the Nightingale Initiative for global health: Florence Nightingale's integral legacy for the 21st century. *Journal of Integral Theory and Practice. 6*(4).

Bentz, V. & Shapiro, J. (1998). *Mindful inquiry in social research.* Thousand Oaks, CA: Sage

Berger, J. (2004). Dancing on the threshold of meaning. *Journal of Transformative Education. 2*, 226-351.

Biggerstaff, D. (2012). Qualitative research methods in psychology. *InTech Open Access.* Retrieved from: http://wrap.warwick.ac.uk/45345/1/WRAP_ Biggerstaff_Qualitative _chapter_InTech_amended_March_NO_TC_revised_V3_Feb_2012_submitted.pdf

Bleakley, A. (2000). Writing with invisible ink: Narrative, confessionalism and reflective practice. *Reflective Practice. 1*(1), 11-24.

Bleakley, A. (2005). Stories as data, data as stories: Making sense of narrative inquiry in clinical education. *Medical Education.*

Booth, M. (2015). *Cannabis: A history.* Los Angeles: MacMillan.

Boyd, R. & Myers, J. (1988). Transformative education. *International Journal of Lifelong Education. 7*(4), 261-284.

Brewer, M. & Gardner, W. (1996). Who is this "we"? Levels of collective identity and self-representation. *Journal of Personality and Social Psychology. 71*(1), 83.

Bruner, J. (1986). *Actual minds, possible worlds*. Cambridge, MA: Harvard University Press.

Burns, J. M. (1978). *Leadership*. New York: Harper & Row.

Charon, R. (1993). The narrative road to empathy. In: Spiro, H., Curnen, M., Peschel, E., & St. James, D., *Empathy and the practice of medicine: Beyond pills and the scalpel*. New Haven, Conn: Yale University Press.

Charon, R. (2006). *Narrative medicine: Honoring the stories of illness*. New York City: Oxford University Press.

Clandinin, D. & Connelly, F. (2000). Narrative Inquiry. *The Sage encyclopedia of qualitative research methods*. 542-545.

Clark, M. & Wilson, A. (1991). Context and rationality in Mezirow's theory of transformational learning. *Adult Education Quarterly. 41*, 75-91.

Colorado Department of Public Health. (2013, December). Medical marijuana registry program update. Retrieved from: https://www.colorado.gov/pacific/sites/default/files/CHED_MMJ_12_2013_MMR_report.pdf

Colorado University School of Medicine. (2016, September 21) Difficulties studying medical marijuana. Retrieved from: http://www.ucdenver.edu/academics/colleges/medicalschool/administration/news/ResearchNews/Pages/Challenges-to-Medical-Marijuana-Research.aspx

Commons, M., et. al. (1990). *Adult development volume 2: Models and methods in the study of adolescent and adult thought*. New York: Praeger Publishing.

Compton, E. (2014). *Disparately deviant labor: From marijuana dealers to marijuana doctors. (Doctoral dissertation)*. Wesleyan University.

Corbin, T., et. al. (2011). Developing a trauma-informed emergency department-based intervention for victims of urban violence. *Journal of Trauma & Dissociation. 12*(5), 510-525.

Cragg, C., Plornikoff, R., Hugo, K., & Casey, A. (2001). Perspective transformation over time: A two-year follow-up study of HIV positive adults. *Adult Education Quarterly. 48*, 65-84.

Cranton, P. (1994). Understanding and promoting transformative learning: A Guide for educators of adults. *Jossey-Bass Higher and Adult Education Series.* San Francisco: Jossey-Bass.

Creswell, J. & Plano-Clark, V. (2007). *Designing and conducting mixed methods research.* Newbury Park, CA: Sage.

Creswell, J. (2012). *Qualitative inquiry and research design: Choosing among five approaches.* Thousand Oaks, CA: Sage.

Cumming, J. & Cumming, E. (1965). On the stigma of mental illness. *Community Mental Health Journal. 1*(2), 135-143.

Datta, A. & Dave, D. (2016). Effects of physician-directed pharmaceutical promotion on prescription behaviors: Longitudinal evidence. *Health Economics.* Doi: 10.1002/hec.3323.

Denzin, N. (1989). *Interpretive biography: Qualitative research methods.* Newbury Park, CA: Sage.

Denzin, N. and Lincoln, Y., Eds. (2000). *Handbook of qualitative research.* Thousand Oaks, CA: Sage.

DeWitt, D., et. al. (2000). The influence of early and frequent use of marijuana on the risk of desistance and the progression of marijuana-related harm. *Preventive Medicine. 31*(5), 455-464.

Earleywine, M. (2002). Understanding marijuana: A new look at the scientific evidence. Oxford: Oxford University Press.

Edwards, M. (2005). The integral holon: A holonomic approach to organizational change and transformation. *Journal of Organizational Change Management. 18*(3), 269-288.

Edwards, M. (2008a). Every today was a tomorrow: An integral method for indexing the social mediation of preferred futures. *Futures. 40*(2), 173-189.

Edwards, M. (2008b). Evaluating integral meta-theory. *Journal of Integral Theory and Practice. 3(4)*, 61-83.

Esbjörn-Hargens, S. (2009). An overview of integral theory: An all-inclusive framework for the 21st century. *Integral Institute. Resource Paper No. 1.* 1-24.

Esbjörn-Hargens, S. Ed. (2010). *Integral theory in action: Applied, theoretical, and constructive perspective on the AQAL model*. New York City: State University of New York Press.

Fine, D. (2014). *Hemp bound: Dispatches from the front lines of the next agricultural revolution*. White River Junction, VT: Chelsea Green Publishing.

Fish, S. (1989). Being interdisciplinary is so very hard to do. *Profession*. 15-22.

Foucault, M. (1990). *The history of sexuality, vol. 1: An introduction*. New York City: Vintage Books.

Freire, P. (1984). *Pedagogy of the oppressed*. New York City: Continuum.

Gauthier, A. & Fowler, M. (2008). Integrally-informed approaches to transformational leadership development. *1st bi-annual Integral Theory Conference*. J.F.K. University, Pleasant Hill, CA.

Gee, J. (2001). Identity as an analytic lens for research in education. *Review of Research in Education*. 25.

Genette, G. (1980). *Narrative discourse: An essay in method*. New York: Cornell University Press.

Green, S., et. al. (2005). Living stigma: The impact of labeling stereotyping, separation, status loss, and discrimination in the lives of individuals with disabilities and their families. *Sociological Inquiry*. 75(2), 197-215.

Greenfield, B., et. al. (2015). Power and promise of narrative for advancing physical therapist education and practice. *Physical Therapy*. 95(6): 924-933.

Greenhalgh, T. & Hurwitz, B. (1998). *Narrative based medicine: Dialogue and discourse in clinical practice*. London: B.M.J. Books.

Greenhalgh, T. (2010). What is this knowledge that we seek to 'exchange'? *Milbank Quarterly*. 88(4), 492-499.

Greenleaf, R. (2002). *Servant leadership: A journey into the nature of legitimate power and greatness*. (Third edition). Mahwah, NJ: Paulist Press.

Gregory, T. & Raffanti, M. (2009). Integral diversity maturity: Toward a postconventional understanding of diversity dynamics. *Journal of Integral Theory and Practice*. 4(3).

Halpern, J. (2001). *From detached concern to empathy: Humanizing medical practice*. New York: Oxford University Press.

Hathaway, A. (2004). Cannabis users informal rules for managing stigma and risk. *Deviant Behavior. 25*(6), 559-577.

Hathaway, A., Comeau, N., & Erickson, P. (2011). Cannabis normalization and stigma: Contemporary practices of moral regulation. *Criminology and Criminal Justice.*

Herer, J. (1998). *The emperor wears no clothes.* Austin, TX: Ah Ha Publishers.

Hersey, P., Blanchard, K., & Natemeyer, W. (1979). Situational leadership, perception, and the impact of power. *Group & Organization Management. 4*(4), 428-428.

House, R. (1996). Path-goal theory of leadership: Lessons, legacy, and a reformulated theory. *The Leadership Quarterly. 7*(3), 323-352.

Howard, H. (1999). *Intelligence reframed: Multiple intelligences for the 21st century.* New York: Basic Books.

Huddleston, Jr., T. (2016). Colorado's legal marijuana industry is worth $1 billion. *Fortune.* Retrieved from: http://fortune.com/2016/02/11/marijuana-billion-dollars-colorado/

Illinois Department of Public Health. (June, 2015). Illinois Medical Cannabis Registry Pilot Program. *Year-end 2015 Report.*

Illinois Department of Public Health. (January, 2016). Illinois Medical Cannabis Registry Pilot Program. *Mid-Year 2016 Report.*

Illinois Department of Public Health. (June, 2016). Illinois Medical Cannabis Registry Pilot Program. *Year-end 2016 Report*

Ingold, J. (2016, July 19). Four Colorado doctors suspended over medical marijuana recommendations. *Denver Post.* Retrieved from: http://www.denverpost.com/2016/07/19/four-colorado-doctors-suspended-over-medical-marijuana-recommendations/

Ingraham, C. (2016, April 15). More and more doctors want marijuana legal. *Washington Post Live.* Retrieved from: https://www.washingtonpost.com/news/wonk/wp/2016/04/15/more-and-more-doctors-want-to-make-marijuana-legal/?utm_term=.ce905b7b5309

Jaywork, C. (2016, July 1). Little drama, lots of doubts as Washington medical marijuana industry goes dark. *Seattle Weekly.* Retrieved from: http://www.seattleweekly.com/news/all-pot-dispensaries-must-be-closed-as-of-today/

Joy, J., Watson, S., & Benson, J., Eds. (1999). *Marijuana and medicine: assessing the science base*. Washington, D.C.: National Academy Press.

Kaplan, A. (2002). *Development practitioners and social process: Artists of the invisible*. London: Pluto Press.

Kaplan, A. (2005). Emerging out of Goethe: Conversation as a form of social inquiry. *Janus Head. 8*(1), 311-334.

Kegan, R. (2000). *Learning as Transformation*. Los Angeles: Jossey-Bass.

Kerr, S. & Jermier, J. (1978). Substitutes for leadership: Their meaning and measurement. *Organizational Behavior and Human Performance. 22*(3), 375-403.

Kietzmann, J., Hermkens, K., McCarty, I., & Silvestre, B. (2016). Social media? Get serious? Understanding the functional building blocks of social media. *Science Direct*. Retrieved from: http://busandadmin.uwinnipeg.ca/silvestrepdfs/PDF06.pdf

Kings, K. (2002). Educational technology professional development as transformative learning opportunities. *Computers & Education. 39*(3), 283-297.

Koestler, A. (1967). *The ghosts in the machine*. London: Hutchinson of London.

Konrad, E. & Reid, A. (2013). Colorado family physicians' attitudes toward medical marijuana. *Journal of American Board of Family Medicine. Jan-Feb*, 52-60.

Koungange, N. (2015). Drug overdose deaths reach all-time high. *CNN*. Retrieved from: http://www.cnn.com/2015/12/18/health/drug-overdose-deaths-2014

Kreisberg, J. (2012). Three principles of integral healthcare. *Explore. 8*(6), 370-372.

Laatscch, L., et. al. (2005). Cooperative learning effects on teamwork attitudes in clinical laboratory science students. *Clinical Laboratory Science. 18*(3), 150-152.

Ladkin, D. (2010). *Rethinking leadership: A new look at old leadership questions*. London. Edward Elgar Publishing.

Lange, E. (2004). Transformative and restorative learning. A vital dialectic for sustainable societies. *Adult Education Quarterly. 54*(2), 121-139.

Leonard, K. (2016, September 15). Study: Opioid use decreased in states that legalize medical marijuana. *U.S. News & World Report*. Retrieved from: http://www.usnews.com/news/articles/2016-09-15/study-opioid-use-decreases-in-states-that-legalize-medical-marijuana

Lieb, K. & Scheurich, A. (2014). Contact between doctors and the pharmaceutical industry, their perceptions and the effects on prescribing habits. *PLoS One*. 10.1371/journal.pone.011013.

Lieberman, A. & Solomon, A. (2008). Cruel choice: Patients forced to decide between medical marijuana and employment. *Hofstra Labor & Employment Law Journal*. *26*, 619.

Liimatainen, L., et. al. (2001). The development of reflective learning in the context of health counselling and health promotion during nurse education. *Journal of Advanced Nursing*. *34*(5), 648-658.

Linn, L., Yager, J., & Leake, B. (1989). Physicians' attitudes toward the legalization of marijuana use. *Western Journal of Medicine*. *150*(6), 714-717.

Lopez, F. (2016, August 5). Public meeting held on medical cannabis card delays. *KRQE*. Retrieved from: http://krqe.com/2016/08/04/public-meeting-planned-over-medical-cannabis-card-delays

Lucas, P. (2012). Cannabis as an adjunct or substitute for opiates in the treatment of chronic pain. *Journal of Psychoactive Drugs*. *44*(2), 125-133.

Lundy, T. (2010). A paradigm to guide health promotions into the 21st century.: The integral idea whose time has come. *Global Health Promotion*. *17*(3), 44-53.

Lynch, M. & Clark, A. (2003). Cannabis reduces opioid dose in the treatment of chronic non-cancer pain. *Journal of Pain and Symptom Management*. *25*(6), 496-498.

Marshall, C. & Rossman, G. (2011). *Designing qualitative research* (5th ed). Thousand Oaks, CA: Sage.

McPartland, J., et. al. (2006). Evolutionary origins of the endocannabinoid system. *Gene*. *370*, 64-74.

Mezirow, J. (1991). *Transformative dimensions of adult learning*. Los Angeles: Jossey-Bass.

Mezirow, J. (1996). Contemporary paradigms of learning. *Adult Education Quarterly*. *46*, 158-172.

Mezirow, J. (2000). *Learning as Transformation*. Los Angeles: Jossey-Bass.

Mikuriya, T., Bearman, D., Hergenrather, J., Lucido, F., Denny, P., & Nunberg, H. (2007). Medical marijuana in California, 1996-2006. *O'Shaughnessy's*, *1*(4), 41-43.

Neimeyer, R. (2004). Construction of death and loss: Evolution of a research program. *Personal Construct Theory and Practice*, *1*, 8-22.

Nelson, R. (2014). *Theorist-at-large: One woman's ambiguous journey into medical cannabis*. Seattle: CreateSpace.

Nelson, R. (2015). *The eCS Therapy Companion Guide*. Seattle: CreateSpace.

Nelson, R. (2016, May 5). AQAL: Untangling an egregious social wrong. *Integral European Conference*. Siofok, Hungary,

Newport, F. (2011). Record-high 50% of Americans favor legalizing marijuana use. Retrieved from: http://www.gallup.com/poll/150149/record-high-americans-favor-legalizing-marijuana.aspx

Northouse, P. (2010). *Leadership: Theory and practice* (5th edition). Los Angeles: Sage.

Nunberg, H., et. al. (2011). An analysis of applicants presenting to a medical marijuana specialty practice in California. *Journal of Drug Policy Analysis. 4*(1).

Nussbaum, A., Boyer, J., & Kondrad, E. (2011). But my doctor recommended pot: Medical marijuana and the patient-physician relationship. *Journal of General Internal Medicine. 26*(1), 1364-1367.

Nutt, D. (2009). Government vs. science over drug and alcohol policy. *The Lancet. 374*, 1731-1733.

Nye, J. (2008). *The powers to lead*. London: Oxford University Press.

O'Brien, P. (2013). Medical marijuana and social control: Escaping criminalization and embracing medicalization. *Deviant Behavior. 34*(6), 423-443.

O'Catherine, A. (2015). New Mexico worker's compensation administration establishes reimbursement process for medical marijuana in work comp cases. *State of New Mexico Worker's Compensation Administration Bulletin, 19*(4).

O'Shea, T. (2001) Conventional medicine vs. holistic medicine. A world of difference. *New West Publications*. Retrieved from: https://www.cancertutor.com/conventional-medicine-vs-holistic-a-world-of-difference/.

Ogborne, A., Smart, R., & Adlaf, E. (2014). Self-reported medical use of marijuana: A survey of the general population. *Canadian Medical Association Journal. 162*(12), 1685-1686.

Pacula, R., Boustaed, A., & Hunt, P. (2014). Words can be deceiving: A review of variation among legally effective medical marijuana laws in the United States. *Journal of Drug Policy Analysis. 7*(1), 1-19.

Paley, J. & Eva, G. (2005). Narrative vigilance: The analysis of stories in health care. *Nursing Philosophy. 6*(2), 83-97.

Paley, J. (2009) Narrative machinery. *Narrative Stories in Health Care, Illness, Dying and Bereavement. 1*, 17-32.

Paley, J. & Lilford, R. (2011). Qualitative methods: An alternative view. *BMJ. 342*, 957-958.

Patton, M. (1990). *Qualitative evaluation and research methods.* Thousand Oaks, CA: Sage.

Patton, M. (2005). *Qualitative research.* Los Angeles: John Wiley & Sons.

Pedersen, W. (2009). Cannabis use: Subcultural opposition or social marginality? A population-based longitudinal study. *Acta Sociologica. 52*(2), 135-148.

Pedersen, W. & Sandberg, S. (2013). The medicalization of revolt: A sociological analysis of medical cannabis users. *Sociology of Health and Illness. 35*(1), 17-32.

Petrie, D. (2011). An integral methodological pluralism framework for evidence-based medicine. *Journal of Integral Theory & Practice. 6*(4).

Petrocellis, L., Grazia Cascio, M., & Di Marzo, V. (2004). The endocannabinoid system: A general view and latest additions. *British Journal of Pharmacology. 141*(5), 765-774.

Polkinghorne, D. (1988). *Narrative knowing and the human sciences.* Albany, NY: State University of New York Press.

Reams, J. (2014). A brief overview of developmental theory or "What I learned in the FOLA Course". *Integral Review. 10*(1).

Reiman, A. (2007). Medical cannabis patients: Patient profiles and health care utilization patterns. *Complementary Health Practice Review. 12*(1), 31-50.

Reiman, A. (2008). Self-efficacy, social support and service integration at medical cannabis facilities in the San Francisco Bay area of California. *Health & Social Care in the Community. 16*(1), 31-41.

Reiman, A. (2009). Cannabis as a substitute of alcohol and other drugs. *Harm Reduction Journal. 6*(1), 2-6.

Reinarman, C., et. al. (2011). Who are medical marijuana patients? Population characteristics from nine California assessment clinics. *Journal of Psychoactive Drugs. 43*(2), 128-135.

Remler, D. & Van Ryzin, G. (2011). *Research methods in practice: Strategies for description and causation.* Los Angeles: Sage.

Richardson, L. (1990). Narrative and sociology. *Journal of Contemporary Ethnography.* *19*(1), 116-120.

Salzet, M. & Stefano, G. (2002). The endocannabinoid system in invertebrates. *Prostaglandins, Leukotrienes, and Essential Fatty Acids.* *66*(2), 353-361.

Say, R., Murtagh, M., & Thomson, T. (2006). Patients preference for involvement in medical decision making: A narrative review. *Patient Education and Counseling.* *60*(2), 102-114.

Schwartz, M. (2010). Frames of AQAL, integral critical theory and the emerging integral arts. *Integral Theory in Action: Applied, Theoretical and Constructive Perspective on the AQAL Model.* *1*, 229-252.

Shamir, B., Dayan-Horesh, H., & Adler, D. (2005). Leading by biography: Towards a life-story approach to the study of leadership. *Leadership.* *4*(3), 110-115.

Shen, L. (2016, May 9). Some people are moving to the U.S. just for medical marijuana. *Fortune Health.* Retrieved from: http://fortune.com/2016/05/09/medical-marijuana-immigration/

Short, B. (2006a). Integral psychiatry: Five elements of clinical theory and practice. *Journal of Integral Theory and Practice.* *1*(2), 113-130.

Short, B. (2006b). Introduction to integral psychiatry. *Journal of Integral Theory and Practice.* *1*(2), 105-112.

Smith, B. (1981). Narrative versions, narrative theories. In Mitchell, W. (ed). *On Narrative.* Chicago, IL: University of Chicago Press.

Smith B., et. al. (2015). Narrative as a knowledge translation tool for facilitating impact: Translating physician activity knowledge to disable people and health professionals. *Health Psychology.* *34*(4), 303-308.

Smucker-Barnwell, S., Earleywine, M., & Wilcox, R. (2006, January 12). Cannabis, motivation, and life satisfaction in an internet sample. *Substance Abuse, Treatment, Prevention, and Policy.* *24*, 169-174.

Strauss, A. & Corbin, J. (1990). *Basics of qualitative research.* Volume 15. Newbury Park, CA: Sage.

Tappan, M. (2010). Telling moral stories: From agency to authorship. *Human Development.* *53*(2), 81-86.

Taylor, E. (1998). Transformative learning: A critical review. *Eric Clearinghouse on Adult, Career, and Vocational Education.* Information Series No. 374.

Teague, C. (2016, June 8). Vulnerable patients in danger from expired medical card delays. Retrieved from: http://herb.co/2016/06/08/danger-expired-medical-card-delays/

Tharp, T. (2008). *The creative habit*. New York City: Simon & Schuster.

Torbert, W. (1991). *The power of balance: Transforming self, society and scientific inquiry*. Newbury Park, CA: Sage.

Torbert & Associates. (2004). *Action inquiry: The secret of timely and transforming leadership*. San Francisco: Barrett-Koehler.

Vance, B. (2016, January 21). Big changes to come to Oregon cannabis industry this year. *Oregon Public Broadcasting*. Retrieved from: http://www.opb.org/news/article/marijuana-cannabis-oregon-recreational-sales-laws/

Vickers, A. & de Craen, A. (2000). Why use placebos in clinical trials? A narrative review of the methodological literature. *Journal of Clinical Epidemiology. 53*(2), 157-161.

Volckmann, R. (2012). Integral leadership and diversity: Definitions, distinctions and implications. *Integral Leadership Review. 12*(3), 1-21.

Vroom, V. & Yetton, P. (1973). *Leadership and decision-making*. Vol. 10. Pittsburgh, PA: University of Pittsburgh Press.

Walsh, R. & Reams, J. (2015). Studies of wisdom: A special issue of integral review. *Integral Review. 11*(2).

Wheatley, M. (2007). A new paradigm for new leadership. In Cuoto, R., Ed. *Reflections on Leadership*. Lanham, MD: University Press of America. 105-115.

Wilber, K. (1995). *Sex, ecology, spirituality: The spirit of evolution*. Boston: Shambala.

Wilber, K. (1996). A brief history of everything. Boston: Shambala.

Wilber, K. (2000a). *Integral psychology: Consciousness, spirit, psychology, therapy*. Boston: Shambala.

Wilber, K. (2000b). *A theory of everything: An integral vision for business, politics, science and spirituality*. Boston: Shambala.

Wilber, K. (2013). *The integral approach: A short introduction by Ken Wilber*. ISBN: 9780834829060. Boston: Shambala.

Williams, D. & Garner, J. (2002). The case against 'the evidence': A different perspective on evidence-based medicine. *The British Journal of Psychiatry. 180*(1), 8-12.

Willig, C. (2013). *Introducing qualitative research in psychology*. London: McGraw-Hill Education.

Young, S. (2014, March 10). Medical marijuana refugees: This was our only hope. *CNN Health*. Retrieved from: http://www.cnn.com/2014/03/10/health/medical-marijuana-refugees/

Ziemianski, D., et. al. (2015) Cannabis in medicine: A national educational needs assessment among Canadian physicians. *BMC Medical Education*. 15, 52-58.

Zucker, D. (2011). An inquiry into integral medicine. *Journal of Integral Theory and Practice* 6(4), 131-136.

Please consider supporting Dr. Nelson's ongoing work:

www.MyECSTherapy.ORG

www.IntegralEducationandConsulting.COM

73762103R00140

Made in the USA
Columbia, SC
17 July 2017

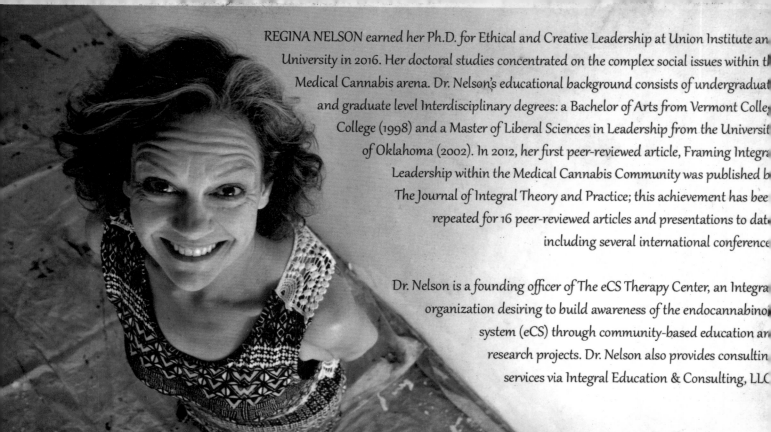

REGINA NELSON earned her Ph.D. for Ethical and Creative Leadership at Union Institute an[d] University in 2016. Her doctoral studies concentrated on the complex social issues within t[he] Medical Cannabis arena. Dr. Nelson's educational background consists of undergraduat[e] and graduate level Interdisciplinary degrees: a Bachelor of Arts from Vermont Colle[ge] College (1998) and a Master of Liberal Sciences in Leadership from the Universit[y] of Oklahoma (2002). In 2012, her first peer-reviewed article, Framing Integra[l] Leadership within the Medical Cannabis Community was published b[y] The Journal of Integral Theory and Practice; this achievement has bee[n] repeated for 16 peer-reviewed articles and presentations to dat[e] including several international conference[s]

Dr. Nelson is a founding officer of The eCS Therapy Center, an Integra[l] organization desiring to build awareness of the endocannabino[id] system (eCS) through community-based education an[d] research projects. Dr. Nelson also provides consultin[g] services via Integral Education & Consulting, LLC

IntegralEducationAndConsulting.co[m]
MyECSTherapy.OR[G]

"In witnessing the aghast and awed comments of the University staff - and sizable audience from across the academi[c] spectrum - following Dr. Nelson's online dissertation defense, it was clear to all that she had struck a curious nerve; illuminating a societal injustice of such magnitude and shame, one which those outside the long suffering patient community have little or no concept of."

-Michael Edward Browning, Founding Director, Cinebis Film Institu[te]

Talk with Your Doctor - Talk with Your Patient

Whether your interest in this subject is for
yourself, a patient, or a loved one,
reading this book will help to arm you
(intellectually & emotionally) for the conversation
you have with your patient or healthcare provider.
Get prepared. Then share this book!

MEDICAL / Physician & Patient   © 2017   Author photo: Sharon Letts   Cover design: Michael Browning   **$27.99 US**

VOLUME DISCOUNTS
for nonprofit, clinical or patient organizations
720.767.2047

ISBN 9780975890035
9780975 890035